SPORTS NUTRITION
The Scientific Facts

SPORTS NUTRITION
The Scientific Facts

VAIJAYANTHI V. KANABUR

KANISHKA PUBLISHERS, DISTRIBUTORS
NEW DELHI-110 002

KANISHKA PUBLISHERS, DISTRIBUTORS
4697/5-21A, Ansari Road, Daryaganj
New Delhi -110 002
Phones : 2327 0497, 2328 8285
Fax : 011-2328 8285
E-mail : kanishka_publishing@yahoo.co.in

First Published 2007

Edition–2020

ISBN : 978-81-7391-969-5

PRINTED IN INDIA

Published by Madan Sachdeva for Kanishka Publishers, Distributors, 4697/5-21A, Ansari Road, Daryaganj, New Delhi-110 002, Typeset by Sunshine Graphics, Delhi, and Printed at Rajdhani Printers, Delhi.

Introduction

"All work and no play makes Jack a dull boy" is an age-old saying. Today's Jacks don't have to play just for recreation. Sports and games are no longer thought of as mere entertainment. A number of youngsters are pursuing sports as a career. With the emergence of commercial sponsorship and encouraging support from the government, sports as a profession is gaining popularity.

Even while fully appreciating the true spirit of participation in games and sports, one yet tends to assess performance in terms of success attained through medals and prizes. The crucial factors that influence the athletic performance are physique and physical fitness. Nutrition has a key role to play in determining the physique of a person. However, it is to be noted that without hard work and a strong urge to win, even the best diet would not result in improved performance. It is said, if you think you can, you will. If you think you cannot you will not. But sound nutrition does provide the foundation on which each sports person needs to put the bricks and mortar of innate talent, hard training and a strong drive to excel. Knowing how to put these together produces a champion.

Many champions like Lasse Viren, the Olympic champion of 5000 and 10,000 m in 1972 and 1976 have attributed their achievement to nutritional management (Garrow and James, 1993). It is a fact that many athletes suffer from failure of performance, which may be due to a variety of causes of which dietary factors are easier to remedy.

To understand the importance of nutrition for a sports person, one has to know the basics of the science of nutrition and the physiological effect of physical activity.

AUTHOR

Contents

Contents

1

A, B, C of Nutrition

The word nutrition is derived from a Latin root 'Nutr' meaning to nurture or nourish. Nourishment is that which sustains life. The art and science of human nutrition focuses on nourishing human beings. Food contains chemical substances called nutrients, which perform a variety of physiological functions. There are about 40 essential nutrients required by the human body for maintaining normal health. Food is the vehicle for these nutrients. So nutrition may be defined as food at work. It includes everything that happens to the food from the time it is eaten until it is digested and metabolized. In simple words nutrition deals with what to eat, how much to eat, what not to eat, what happens when we eat in excess or when we eat less or when we do not eat.

Food is necessary for growth, development and to lead an active and healthy life. Human beings have access to a wide range of foods and all foods are not of same quality from nutritional point of view. So the ability to meet the nutritional needs and maintain good health depends upon the type and quantity of foodstuffs included in the diet. Though food is eaten primarily to satisfy hunger, the choice of food is influenced by food availability, purchasing power, socio-cultural factors, emotional factors and personal likes and dislikes. A diet should be planned on sound nutritional principles, without undermining the above factors. Therefore, basic knowledge of food and nutrition is absolutely necessary to make wise decisions regarding food. The nutrients that are necessary for human beings are carbohydrates, proteins, fats, vitamins, minerals and water. Carbohydrates, proteins and fats yield energy whereas vitamin minerals and water do not give any energy. Each nutrient has got its own specific function in the body.

Energy Yielding Nutrients

There are 3 energy yielding nutrients namely, carbohydrates, fats and proteins.

Carbohydrates

Carbohydrates are composed of carbon, hydrogen and oxygen. The carbohydrate family consists of:

I. *Simple Carbohydrates:* These are further divided into:
(a) Monosaccharides (Those containing single sugar units). Example : Glucose, Fructose and Galactose.

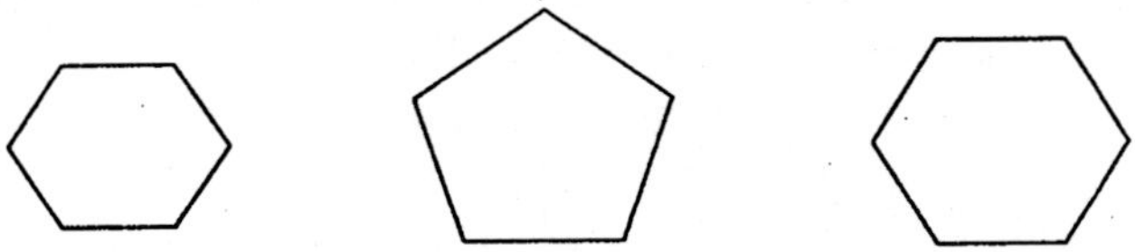

Glucose Fructose Galactose

(b) Disaccharides: Contain a pair of monosaccharides. E.g. Sucrose, Lactose, Maltose.

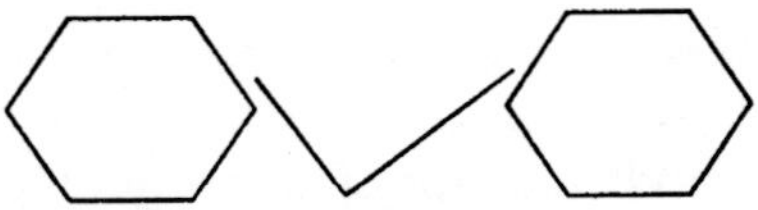

Maltose (Glucose + Glucose)

Lactose

(Glucose + Galactose)

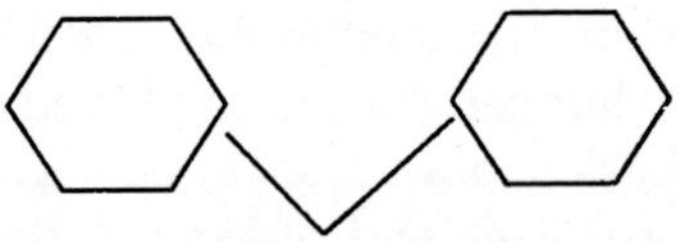

Sucrose

(Glucose + Fructose)

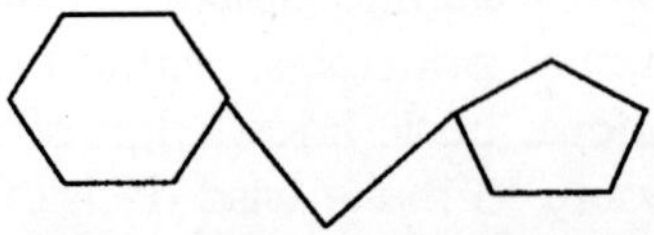

(c) Oligosaccharides: Contain few units of monosaccharides

II. *Complex Carbohydrates:* These contain many units of simple sugars.

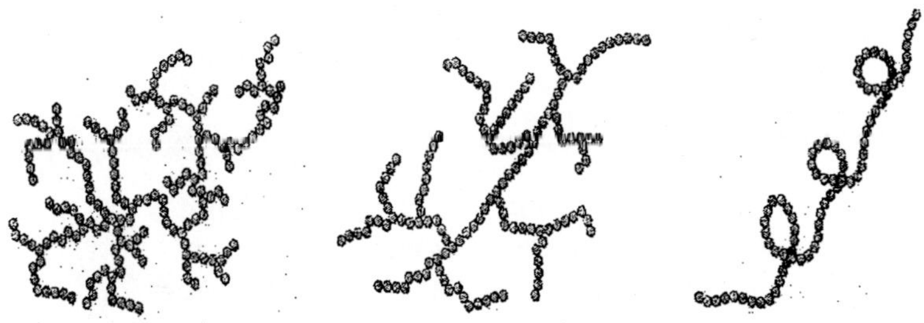

Glycogen Starch (unbranched)

Example: Glycogen is a polymer of glucose. Starch is also made up of many units of glucose. Glycogen is a storage form of carbohydrate in case of animals whereas starch is a storage form of carbohydrate in case of plants. Dietary fiber refers to a group of complex carbohydrates, which are of special significance in human nutrition though they cannot be digested by the human digestive system. Example: Cellulose, hemicellulose, pectin, lignin, gums. These are present in all plant based foods e.g. vegetables, fruits, whole grains, etc. Dietary fibers delay and retard absorption of carbohydrates and fats. So a high fiber diet prevents a rapid rise in post prandial blood glucose level. Experiments have shown that dietary fiber reduces cholesterol in blood, prevents constipation, reduces the risk of colon cancer and is important for diabetic patients.

Functions of Carbohydrates

1. *Source of energy:* Carbohydrate provides 4 Kcal/g of energy. In an Indian diet which is predominantly cereal based almost 60-70 per cent of energy comes from carbohydrates.
2. Carbohydrates exert a protein sparing action. The main function of protein is to provide for growth. In case if adequate energy is not available, the body utilizes protein for energy instead of growth. This results in retardation of growth. When an adequate amount of energy is provided in the form of carbohydrates and fats, then body uses carbohydrates and fat for energy and spares the proteins

for growth. Meeting energy needs takes the first priority over growth.

3. Carbohydrates are essential for the utilization of fat. For complete oxidation of fat oxalic acid is needed. Oxalic acid is an intermediary product of carbohydrate metabolism. If carbohydrates are not provided in adequate amount then the body cannot utilize fat also. That is why it is said "fats burn in the flame of carbohydrates."
4. Carbohydrates are a source of dietary fiber.

Source

Simple carbohydrates like glucose, fructose are found in fruits, honey, vegetables, sucrose in sugar, lactose in milk, polysaccharides like starch are found in cereals, millets, pulses, roots and tubers and glycogen in animal foods. Dietary fiber is found in fruits, leafy vegetables, whole grains and legumes.

Deficiency

1. If adequate amounts of carbohydrates are not consumed, it directly affects the work efficiency and the person will have low vitality.
2. In case of carbohydrate deficiency, proteins will be utilized for energy and this results in protein deficiency.

Proteins: People commonly associate protein with strength and meat with protein. Consequently, they think eating meat builds their muscles. This is only partially correct because proteins are primary structural and functional components of every living cell. Almost half the protein in our body is in the form of muscles and the rest of it is in bone, cartilage and skin.

Chemically proteins are made up of amino acids. Amino acids are made up of carbon, hydrogen, oxygen and nitrogen.

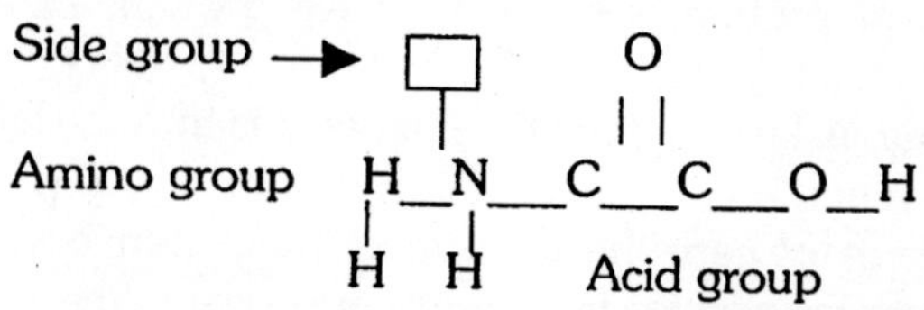

Amino acids are the building blocks of proteins.

–+—Amino acid—Amino acid —Amino acid—sAmino acid—Amino acid—+ —-

Protein

In addition to these, sometimes other elements like sulphur are present in some amino acids.

Some amino acids cannot be synthesized by the human body and therefore have to be supplied from the diet. These are termed as essential amino acids. Other amino acids, can be synthesized by the body they are called non-essential amino acids.

Functions

1. Proteins are necessary for growth and maintenance. They form integral part of most body structures such as tendons, membranes, muscles, organs and bones. Wherever the body is growing, repairing or replacing the tissue, proteins are involved.
   From the moment of conception, as the baby grows it uses proteins as building blocks. E.g. to build a bone or a tooth, cells first lay down a matrix of protein collagen and then fill it with crystals of calcium, phosphorus, fluoride and other minerals. The protein collagen is also the material of ligaments and tendons and the strengthening glue between the cells. The scars that knit the separated parts of torn tissues are made up of collagen protein.
   As old skin cells fall off, new cells made largely of proteins grow from underneath to compensate. Cells in the deeper skin layers synthesize new proteins to go into hair and fingernails. Digestive tract cells are replaced every 3 days. So body constantly deposits protein into new cells that replace the dead, worn out cells.
2. All enzymes are proteins. Enzymes are nothing but biocatalysts. Thus proteins facilitate chemical reactions in the body.
3. Proteins regulate body processes in the form of hormones.
4. Antibodies, which protect the body against the diseases, are made up of proteins.
5. Proteins help in fluid and electrolyte balance, i.e., proteins

help to maintain the fluid volume and the composition of body fluids.

6. Proteins act as buffers (They resist the change in the P^H and help in maintaining the acid base balance of body fluids.
7. Proteins help in transportation of lipids, vitamins, minerals, and oxygen around the body.
8. Proteins also provide energy. 1 gram provides 4 Kcal of energy. Providing energy is not the primary function of proteins. If there is a deficiency of energy from other sources (Carbohydrates and fats), then proteins will be used for energy.

Sources

Plant foods like legumes; animal foods like milk, meat, fish and eggs are rich sources of protein. The protein content of some common foods is as follows.

Rice: 6-7%
Wheat: 11-12%
Maize: 4%
Jowar:10.4%
Bajra:11.6%
Bengal gram: 18-20%
Black gram: 24%
Peas (dry): 20%
Red gram: 22%
Soyabean: 43.2%
Leafy vegetables: 1-5%
Roots and tubers: 0-1%
Nuts and oilseeds: 20-25%
Fruits Negligible.
Fish and sea foods: 15-20%
Meat: 18-20%
Egg: 12-13%
Cow's Milk: 3.2%
Buffalo Milk: 4.3%
Cheese 24%
Skimmed milk powder: 38%
Whole milk power: 25.8%

The foods differ not only in the quantity of proteins but also the quality of proteins. One of the methods of evaluating protein quality is by analyzing amino acid composition. If a dietary protein contains all essential amino acids in adequate amounts then it is referred to as complete protein. E.g. egg, milk, meat, fish, etc.

Mutual Supplementation of Proteins

Generally proteins derived from animals such as meat, fish, poultry, egg, milk are complete proteins as they contain all essential amino acids. But this does not mean that vegetarians have to consume animal proteins to meet their protein needs. Vegetarians can consume two or more proteins whose amino acid composition is such that the essential amino acid missing from one are supplied by the other. This is known as mutual supplementation of proteins. Example, cereals in general lack lysine and threonine, while legumes, milk, fish and meat are good sources of these amino acids. Legumes lack sulphur containing amino acids (Methionine) and tryptophan, which are present in good amounts in cereal proteins. So a combination of cereals and pulses brings the complementary proteins together. Example, idli, wheat bread and peanut butter, rice/chapati with sprouted pulses.

Deficiency

Deficiency of proteins can have devastating effect on health. In case of children it leads to growth retardation and in case of adults weight loss and wasting of muscles.

Lipids

The lipid family consists of (1) *Triglycerides*—Each triglyceride consists of one molecule of glycerol and 3 molecules of fatty acids.

Fatty acid + Fatty acid + Fatty acid + Glycerol ⟶ Glycerol (— Fatty acid, — Fatty acid, — Fatty acid)

Triglyceride

Fatty acids may be saturated (when only single bonds are present) or unsaturated (when one or more double bonds are present). If they have more than one double bond then they are known as Poly Unsaturated Fatty Acids (PUFA). PUFA are of special interest in human nutrition as they regulate blood pressure, clotting and other body functions important to health.

(2) Phospholipids: E.g. Lecithin.
(3) Sterols: E.g. Cholesterol.

Functions

1. Lipids are a concentrated source of energy. 1g of lipid gives 9 Kcal whereas same quantity of carbohydrate or protein provides only 4 Kcal.
2. Lipids are essential for absorption of Vitamins A, D, E, K and carotenoids (Precursors of Vitamin A). Fats serve as vehicles for fat soluble vitamins and promote their absorption.
3. Fats provide essential fatty acids, which are necessary for normal health.
4. They reduce the bulk of the diet, improve the palatability and give satiety value (a feeling of fullness in the stomach).
5. Fats stored in the adipose tissue act as a reserve form of energy during starvation, illness etc.
6. Phospholipids are an important constituent of cell membrane, helps in transport of fat and cholesterol, blood coagulation and normal functioning of nervous system.
7. Cholesterol plays an important role in the formation of bile acids (which are necessary for digestion of lipids), necessary for maintaining the cell membrane, precursor of steroid hormones, Vitamin D etc.

Source

Most lipids are a mixture of saturated, monounsaturated and poly unsaturated fatty acids. The single most important factor as far as fats are concerned is the degree of saturation. Generally speaking, if they are saturated, they are solid at room temperature. If they are unsaturated they are liquid at room temperature (oils). In general lipids of plant origin are poly unsaturated e.g. vegetable oil. There are two exceptions to this palm oil, coconut oil. Animal fats are usually saturated fats, e.g., butter, margarine.

Vegetable oils such as olive oil, canola oil, peanut oil, are rich in mono unsaturated oil. Safflower oil, sunflower oil, corn oil, soyabean oil are rich in PUFA. Coconut oil, butter, beef, tallow and palm oil are rich in saturated fats.

Sources of Essential Fatty Acids

Omega 6 linoleic acid: Leafy vegetables, seeds, nuts, grains, vegetable oil.

Arachidonic acid: Meat or can be made from linoleic acid.

Omega 3 linolenic acid: Fats and oils (Canola, soyabean, wheat germ, margarine), Nuts and seeds (Butternuts, soyabean kernals), Vegetable (soyabean), fish.

Cholesterol Content of Foods

Interestingly cholesterol is present only in foods of animal origin. Cholesterol content of foods is as follows:

Foods	*Cholesterol mg/100 g*
Dairy Products	
Butter	280
Ghee	310
Cheese, Swiss processed	145
Cheese, American processed	160
Cream processed	140
Milk, whole (fresh)	11
Milk, skimmed (fresh)	0.1
Milk, powder (whole)	8
Milk, powder (skimmed)	0.4
Poultry Products	
Egg, Hen (whole)	498
Egg, yolk	1330
Egg, white	0
Egg, chicken, dark	60
Egg, whole (dried)	3900
Flesh Foods	
Beef, round lean	95
Beef, round medium fat	125
Duck	70

(Contd.)

Foods	*Cholesterol mg/100 g*
Lamb	70
Pigeon	110
Pork	60
Rabbit	50
Veal	100
Beef, liver	260
Calf, liver	360
Lamb, liver	610
Pork, liver	420
Brain	2000
Heart	150
Kidney	375
Animal Fat	
Lard and other animal fats	95
Fish and Sea Foods	
Cod	50
Crab	145
Frog	40
Lobster	200
Mackerel	80
Oysters	200
Sardine	70
Shrimps	150
Tuna	65

Vitamins

Carbohydrates, proteins, fats play a leading role in the body. Vitamins and minerals are their supporting cast. Chemically vitamins are the organic compounds required in small amounts to perform specific functions that promote growth, reproduction or the maintenance of health. The word vitamin is derived from a Latin word Vita meaning life and amine means a class of chemical compounds. Though vitamins are needed in very small amounts–micrograms or milligrams but the role played by them is very important. They act as co-enzymes and co-factors in metabolism. They do not provide any calorie but are necessary for the release of energy, e.g. thiamin (Vitamin B_1) is necessary for the metabolism of carbohydrates. Each vitamin has got its own specific function. The role of each vitamin is briefly discussed below:

Vitamins are broadly classified into 2 groups:

1. Fat soluble vitamins —A, D, E and K.
2. Water soluble vitamins—B complex and C.

Vitamin A

Vitamin A is a pale yellow substance found in 2 forms. Vitamin A and Carotenoids. Carotenoids are the precursors of Vitamin A (can be converted into Vitamin A in the body). But the efficiency of conversion is low. Vitamin A is involved in many functions:

1. It is necessary for normal vision.
2. It plays a role in cell growth and development of healthy skin and hair.
3. It is necessary for bone growth and tooth development in children.
4. Vitamin A helps to fight against infections.
5. It is essential for maintaining the protective lining of lungs, stomach, intestine, urinary tract, reproductive system.
6. It is necessary for normal reproduction and some studies have shown that Vitamin A reduces the risk of colon cancer.

Sources

Vitamin A is found only in animal foods such as liver, kidney, butter, cream, whole milk, fish liver oil etc. Vitamin A can be synthesized in the liver from Beta-carotene found in yellow coloured fruits and vegetables (carrots, apricots, mango, papaya). Intensely green leafy vegetables also contain carotene e.g. drumstick, spinach, fenugreek leaves, curry leaves etc. To get enough Vitamin A, it is recommended to consume a dark green, deep orange fruit or vegetable at least every alternate day. Body has the capacity to store excess Vitamin A in liver, kidney and adipose tissue; carotene stored under the skin gives a glowing colour. That is why a daily glass of fresh vegetable juice helps to get a good complexion.

Even when fruits and vegetables are carefully selected for their green and yellow colour, much of the valuable carotene may not reach the blood because carotene is held inside the cell and walls of the cells are made up of cellulose which cannot be digested by human beings. Many nutrients, which are not soluble in water, can pass through the cell walls of the cellulose but carotene which dissolves only in fat cannot. So unless the cell walls are cut, softened or broken by mechanical means, the carotene is not freed and cannot pass into the blood, e.g., recent research has shown that only 1 per cent of the carotene is absorbed from raw carrots compared to about 30 per cent from cooked carrots. So one has to chew the foods thoroughly or supplement the diet with juice of fresh vegetables, extracted with a juicer, which mashes the cellulose and frees the carotene from the cells.

Since Vitamin A is twice valuable as carotene, it is better to consume the sources of Vitamin A such as liver, kidney, heart and brain. Fish liver oil is known for its Vitamin A. This can be consumed in the form of oil, tablets/capsules.

Vitamin D

Vitamin D, also called sunshine vitamin unlike other vitamins can be synthesized in the body in presence of sunlight. If one has a well-shaped head, harmonious contours of face and features, strong white teeth, rounded chest and straight beautiful legs, the probabilities are that he/she has enjoyed adequate quantities of Vitamin D from infancy.

Vitamin D is essential for proper utilization of calcium as Vitamin D helps in maintaining blood calcium levels and makes sure that there is enough calcium for building bones and teeth. Calcium is necessary for contraction and relaxation of muscles and in nerve transmission. Vitamin D makes sure that calcium is available for these functions.

Sources

Vitamin D is present in liver egg yolk, fish liver oil. Except these few foods, only a small amount of Vitamin D is found in foods. That is why, milk is usually fortified with Vitamin D. When ultraviolet rays fall on the skin, a cholesterol-like compound is converted into Vitamin D and absorbed into the blood.

Vitamin E

No single food factor has provoked such interest as that of Vitamin E. It is known that Vitamin E is necessary for normal reproduction in animal species. It is an excellent antioxidant. It prevents the oxidation of unsaturated fatty acids in the cell membrane and DNA. In the absence of antioxidants, free radicals may destroy the cells (possibly increasing the risk of cancer). Vitamin E is also important for normal red blood cells and white blood cells. Although there have been numerous claims of miraculous things that Vitamin E can do such as delay aging, there is little or no proof of any wondrous results.

Vitamin E is widely distributed in plant foods. Wheat germ oil is the richest source oatmeal, olive oil, corn, whole wheat, legumes, nuts seeds and green leafy vegetables also contain Vitamin E.

Vitamin K

K stands for the Danish word Koagulation (coagulation or clotting). Vitamin K plays an important role in blood clotting (at least 13 different proteins and calcium are involved in blood clotting. Vitamin K is essential for the synthesis of at least 4 of these proteins).

Vitamin K can be synthesized by the bacteria present in the human intestine. It is also present in green leafy vegetables such as spinach, cabbage, chard, kale, carrot tops are also rich in Vitamin K. Since Vitamin K is not harmed by heat or oxygen, the foods can be used either cooked or raw.

Water Soluble Vitamins

Vitamins B complex and C are soluble in water and therefore can be easily absorbed transported. Since they are soluble in water and not in fat, they cannot be stored in the body. Therefore, water-soluble vitamins must be consumed regularly. Water-soluble vitamins must be consumed regularly. Water-soluble vitamins leach into water when foods are boiled/blanched. Cooking methods that require little or no water such as steaming and microwave heating can better retain water-soluble vitamins.

B Complex Vitamins

Vitamin B is not one rather it is a family of 14 or more members. That is why it is often referred to as "B complex" vitamin. The members are thiamin (B_1), riboflavin(B_2), niacin, pyridoxine(B_6), pantothenic acid, folic acid, Vitamin B12 (Cyanocobalamin), biotin etc.

Despite advertisements that claim otherwise, the vitamins are not fuels that give energy. The energy yielding nutrients—carbohydrates, proteins and fats are used for fuel and the Vitamin B helps the body to use that fuel. It is true that without B vitamins, the body would lack energy. Many of the B vitamins serve as coenzymes to the enzymes that release energy from carbohydrate, fat, and protein (coenzyme helps the enzyme to carry out its function. In the absence of the coenzyme, the enzyme cannot function). Thus deficiency of B vitamins directly affects the metabolism. Each member of the B complex family has got its own specific function. These are discussed briefly:

B_1/Thiamine

B_1 in the form of thiamine pyrophosphate (TPP) acts as a coenzyme in the carbohydrate metabolism. It plays an important role in release of energy from carbohydrates. That is why B_1 is important in making a person energetic and helps in preventing fatigue. In addition, it helps in the normal functioning of nervous system and heart.

Rice polish, wheat germ and dried yeast are rich sources of thiamine whereas whole cereals, pulses, oilseeds and nuts are good sources. Fair sources include milled cereals, vegetables, milk, fruits, meat, fish etc.

Riboflavin (B_2)

Like thiamine, riboflavin in the form of FMN (Riboflavin mononucleotide), FAD (Riboflavin dinucleotide) acts as a coenzyme in carbohydrate metabolism. It also supports normal vision and skin health.

Sources

Significant sources of riboflavin include milk, yogurt, cheese, meat, leafy vegetables, whole grain and yeast. The type of yeast important from nutritional point of view is brewer's yeast. Different species of yeast produce different compounds. Yeast cells used in brewing produce alcohol proteins and B vitamins as they grow. The nutrients are removed from beer and wine in the filtering process. Yeast cells used in baking produce mostly CO_2, which causes bread dough to rise.

Vitamin pills in general give thiamine, riboflavin, niacin, pantothenic acid and B_6. While they are excellent for supplementary purposes, they should not be relied upon. Never, Never can such tablets or capsules take the place of natural vital foods. Light can destroy riboflavin, that is why milk is seldom sold in transparent glass or plastic containers. Riboflavin is stable to heat, so cooking does not destroy it.

Niacin

Niacin in the form of NAD (Nicotinamide Adenine Dinucleotide) and NADP (Nicotinamide Adenine Dinucleotide Phosphate) acts as a coenzyme in about 35 reactions. In simple words niacin helps in the utilization of carbohydrates and thus helps in the release of energy from carbohydrates. It is also essential for the normal functioning of the skin, intestinal tract and the nervous system.

Rich sources of niacin include dried yeast, liver, rice polish, peanut (ground nut), whereas whole cereals, legumes, meat and fish are good sources. Tryptophan, an amino acid present in the dietary proteins can be converted into niacin in the human body (about 60mg of tryptophan can yield 1mg niacin). Thiamin, riboflavin, niacin all help release energy, the need for these vitamins increases as calorie needs increase.

Vitamin B_6 (Pyridoxin)

Vitamin B_6 acts as a co-enzyme in carbohydrate, protein and fat metabolism in making and breaking down amino acids. It is also necessary for the synthesis of red blood cells. Rich sources of B_6 are dried yeast, rice polish, wheat germ and liver. Good sources include whole cereals, legumes, nuts and oilseeds, egg, milk, meat, fish, green leafy vegetables.

Pantothenic Acid

Pantothenic acid in the form of coenzyme A (CoA) which participates in a large number of reactions in the metabolism of carbohydrates and fats. It is also necessary for hemoglobin synthesis, cholesterol synthesis.

Rich sources of pantothenic acid are dried yeast, liver (ox, sheep, goat), rice polishings and wheat germ. Good sources of pantothenic acid include whole cereals, peanuts, legumes, milk, meat, egg and leafy vegetables.

Biotin (Anti-Egg White Injury Factor)

Biotin plays an important role in maintaining skin structure and nervous system. It acts as a coenzyme in fatty acid metabolism. Rich sources of Biotin are dry yeast, rice polish, liver and groundnut. Biotin is present in the egg white. But a protein called avidin present in egg combines with biotin and makes it unavailable to the body. When heated, avidin gets destroyed. That is why consumption of raw egg can induce biotin deficiency whereas consumption of cooked egg does not cause biotin deficiency.

Folic Acid

The word 'Folic acid' is derived from the word 'folium' which means leaf. Folic acid is necessary for the maturation of RBC. Folate is a component of enzymes required to form DNA, the genetic material that appears within every body cell. Folate is therefore needed to make new cells. Studies have also shown that folic acid is necessary for normal reproduction, hair growth and healthy skin. Excellent sources of folate include green leafy vegetables, organ meats such as liver, kidney, legumes and orange juice. Good sources include meats, poultry, fish, whole grain bread etc. But folic acid is soluble in water, unstable to heat and destroyed by light. Therefore much of the folate present in the food is lost during cooking and so fresh and lightly cooked foods provide more folic acid.

Vitamin B_{12}

Cyanocobalamin is the chemical name of B_{12}. It is necessary for the maturation of RBC. It is also necessary for carbohydrate, protein and fat metabolism. It is necessary for normal functioning of nervous system. Vitamin B_{12} is found only in foods of animal origin—meat, fish, eggs, milk and milk products. Pure vegetarians who do not consume milk and egg need to include fortified soy milk in their diet.

Choline

Choline plays an important role in nerve impulse transmission. It is a component of phospholipids, which are necessary for the transport of fatty acids and cholesterol. In case of choline deficiency, the fatty acids and cholesterol transport is affected and so they accumulate in the liver. Rich sources of Choline are egg, liver, wheat germ and legumes. Good sources of choline include mutton (lamb, beef, pork), whole cereals, rice polishings, nuts and oil seeds.

Para Amino Benzoic Acid

Studies have shown that PABA is essential for normal growth, normal lactation and for prevention of greying of hair in case of rats. Rich sources of PABA are dried yeast, liver, peanut, wheat germ, etc. There are still several other B vitamins which are not well-understood but are known to be essential to health.

Of all the vital food factors, the B vitamins assume a special importance, because while they may be widely distributed, they are present in very small quantities in the "usual foods". There are 14 recognized members of B family. They do not always occur together, nor do they occur in any definite proportion. Studies have shown that a large percentage of our population is deficient in B complex vitamins. In order to get adequate supply of B vitamins, it is better to get acquainted with the inexpensive wonder food—wheat germ. Wheat germ can be used daily as a cereal, a cooked cereal, in hot cakes, muffins, biscuits, yeast bread, cookies etc. Prefer brown rice to white rice, peanut butter to jams and jellies. Dried brewer's yeast is another wonder food which can be stirred into water, milk, fruit or vegetable juice and can be used daily. People who follow these simple rules usually find that they possess more vigor than they knew was possible.

Vitamin C

Chemically Vitamin C is ascorbic acid. Vitamin C is necessary for the formation of the intercellular substance, which gives elasticity to the body. It plays an important role in collagen formation. (It is also concerned with the formation of the matrix or base of bones, including the dentine of the teeth).

Vitamin C is required for the utilization of certain essential amino acids from proteins, in building and repairing vital tissues, hence Vitamin C helps in the rapid healing of wounds. It is necessary for the maintenance of capillary integrity. It is involved in the development of red blood cells. Ascorbic acid helps to reduce the ferric form of iron (usually foods contain iron in this form). Thus Vitamin C helps in absorption and utilization of dietary iron. Studies have shown that Vitamin C is necessary for cholesterol metabolism. Deficiency of ascorbic acid can lead to a disease called scurvy, which is characterized by general weakness, swollen and tender joints, and hemorrhages bleeding gums and loose teeth.

Some Vitamin C is found in all fresh fruits and vegetables. Richest sources are amla (Indian gooseberry) and guava. Good sources include lime juice, orange, pine apple, mango (ripe), papaya, tomato, green leafy vegetables like drumstick leaves, amaranth leaves, cabbage, sprouted pulses, soaked cereals. It is to be noted that Vitamin C can be easily destroyed by oxidation, heat, alkalies etc. When Vitamin C is exposed to air it is destroyed. During cooking if iron and copper vessels are used, iron and copper act as catalysts and destroy Vitamin C. Since Vitamin C is soluble in water, cutting into fine pieces or washing after cutting also destroy Vitamin C. Adding sodium bicarbonate (soda) to preserve colour during cooking also results in loss of Vitamin C. Frozen foods retain most of their Vitamin C content provided they are put on to cook before being thrown. Dried foods also tend to lose Vitamin C.

It is better to depend largely on raw foods for daily supply. If fresh citrus juice is taken at breakfast, raw vegetables or salads served at lunch and dinner, vegetable juices taken in between the meals or for appetizers and fresh fruit served for desserts, the

Vitamin C needs can easily be met. During infections, fever, arthritis and allergies, after tooth extractions or any type of surgery and when speedy healing is desired larger amounts of Vitamin C rich foods have to be consumed.

Vitamin P (Bioflavonoids)

The letter 'P' is derived from "Permeabilitats-vitamin", or the capillary permeability factor. Capillary permeability refers to the amount of fluid that can pass through a mass of tissue in a given length of time. Vitamin P activity is displayed by a group of plant substances known as 'flavonoids'. Studies have shown that in case of animals, Vitamin P may produce a fall in blood pressure.

It can be said that as long as natural foods are used, one is reasonably sure of getting at least a portion of all the vitamins both known and unknown. When foods are processed, the vitamins and minerals are destroyed during processing. When one considers the many vitamins and their contributions to health, it is easy to see how mistaken people are who believe they can safeguard their health by taking vitamin capsules and eating only the foods their palates dictate. Such capsules contain only a few of the many vitamins now known. And if they are taken, they should be used as a supplement to the diet.

Minerals

Minerals are inorganic elements, which are needed, in small amounts. But they perform important functions like fluid balance—help in maintaining the amount of water in the body, regulate permeability—help to draw chemical substances in and out of the cells, acid base balance—keep blood and tissue fluids from becoming either too acidic or too alkaline. They influence the secretion of glands and are important in sending messages through the nervous system. They also play an important role in contraction and relaxation of muscles. The above mentioned functions are only some of the functions performed. In fact there are 24 minerals necessary for normal functioning of the body. Each mineral has got its own specific role in maintaining the normal health.

The minerals are broadly classified into 2 groups:

1. *Major minerals*: These are essential minerals found in large amounts in the human body (more than 5g). Hence the requirement of these minerals is high.
2. *Minor/Trace minerals*: These minerals are found in smaller amounts in the human body (less than 5g). These are needed in small amounts.

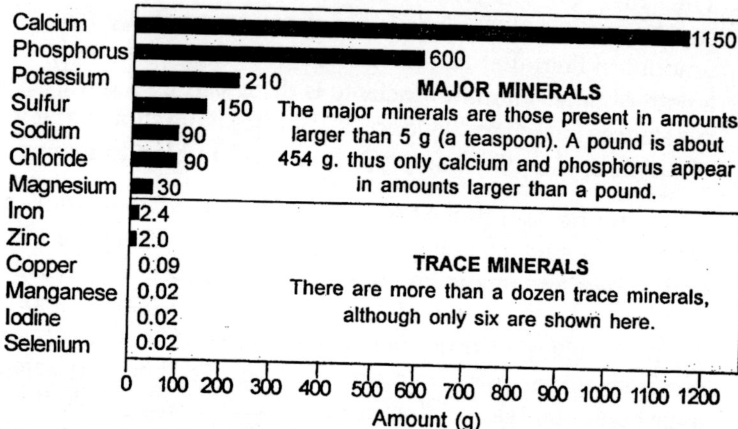

Fig. 1: The Amounts of Minerals in a 60 kg (132-pound) Human Body

Calcium and Phosphorus

Calcium and phosphorous are used for building bones and teeth. These minerals give hardness to the bones and teeth. Calcium helps in muscle contraction and relaxation, contraction of heart, nerve functioning, blood clotting, blood pressure and immune defenses.

Requirement

Adult man—0.4 g/day and growing children 0.6 g/day. For details refer RDA table given in the appendix.

Sources

Richest source is milk (butter milk, skim milk, cheese etc, and green leafy vegetables particularly amaranth, fenugreek and drumstick. Calcium absorption is promoted by lactose (present in milk), Vitamin D (present in milk), presence of phosphorus. Studies have shown that calcium taken with a meal is better absorbed.

Milk and milk products are not only rich in calcium but also in those factors which promote calcium absorption. Unfortunately many people perceive milk as fattening and omit it from their diet in their attempt to lose weight. Instead such people can choose non-fat or low fat milk and milk products. Nutritionists advise daily consumption of 2-3 cups of milk. Teenagers and young adults need 3-4 cups a day.

Those who do not like milk can get their calcium from milk products or milk and milk products can be used as ingredients in preparing other food items. Non-milk sources like some cereals like ragi, small fish with bone, soya milk, almonds etc. can be consumed. It is to be noted that calcium absorption decreases with aging, Vitamin D deficiency, high phosphorus intake, and high fiber diet. Calcium is bound by oxalic acid (present in green leafy vegetables, tea, coffee etc.) and phytates present in whole cereals also makes calcium unavailable to the body. The habit of chewing betel leaves with slaked lime (calcium hydroxide) can also increase calcium intake.

Deficiency

Stunted growth in children as the bones are poorly formed. Bones and teeth become soft and porous. Some bones break easily and teeth lack resistance to decay.

Phosphorus

Calcium and phosphorus are found in the form of calcium phosphate in the bone and teeth. Phosphorus is also involved in the release of energy from carbohydrate, protein and fat (energy currency of the cell is ATP). It is also a constituent of DNA (genetic material). Therefore, it is necessary for growth. It is also constituent of enzymes. Normal processes of the body produce acid and bases that can cause problems to the body. These are neutralized (buffered) by phosphorous.

Requirement

It is said that about a gram of phosphorus should be present in the diet. This amount can be easily obtained even from a poor vegetarian diet (cereal based). So deficiency is rare.

Sources

The rich sources are cereals, pulses, nuts and oilseeds. But 40-80 per cent of phosphorus in these foods occurs in the form of phytin, which is not available to the body. Phosphorus is also present in all animal tissues—meat, fish, poultry, egg and milk.

Sodium and Potassium (Electrolytes)

Sodium, potassium and chloride referred to as electrolytes because when dissolved in the body fluids they separate into positively or negatively charged particles known as ions. Potassium, with a negative charge is found mainly within the cell. Sodium (+ve) ion and chloride ion (-ve) are found in fluid outside the cells.

The electrolytes perform 2 critical balancing acts:

1. *Water balance:* Maintaining the proper amount of water in each of body's 3 compartments i.e., inside the cells, outside the cells and in the blood vessels. Electrolytes maintain the water balance by moving the water around the body.
2. *Acid-base balance:* Electrolytes have the ability to buffer or neutralize various acids and bases in the body. In addition sodium is essential for nerve transmission and muscle contraction.

Sodium Requirement

Sodium is lost in sweat (as NaCl) and in urine. Sodium chloride or common salt not only imparts taste but also provides the necessary amount of sodium required by the body. Salt is about 40 per cent sodium. 1g salt contributes 400mg sodium. 1 tsp = 5 g salt. Therefore 1tsp salt contributes 200mg sodium.

The exact amount of sodium required in a tropical country like India is not known. The daily intake in our diet is as high as 15-20 g/day. Under conditions of excessive sweating as in summer and for those who work in hot environment, a higher intake may be necessary.

Sources of Sodium

As much as 75 per cent of sodium in the diet comes from salt and only a small proportion of sodium comes from natural salt in foods.

In view of association of high blood pressure and salt intake, a lower intake of 8-10 g/day may be advisable. People who have to cut down salt intake may have to avoid highly salted foods and add little or no salt at the table. Foods eaten without salt may seem less tasty but people can learn to enjoy the natural flavour of unsalted foods also. They also have to avoid or reduce consumption of pickles, potato chips, salted popcorn, salted nuts and crackers, cheese-especially processed type.

Deficiency

Vomiting, diarrhoea, heavy sweating can induce sodium deficiency. It can lead to muscle cramps, mental apathy and loss of appetite. If blood sodium drops, both sodium and water must be replenished. Under normal conditions of sweating due to exercise, salt losses can be easily replaced later in the day with ordinary foods. Salt tablets are not recommended because, too much salt with too little water can induce dehydration.

Potassium

Besides maintaining water and electrolyte balance potassium is necessary for nerve transmission and muscle contraction. The exact requirement of potassium is not known but potassium present in a vegetarian diet is probably adequate to meet the daily requirement. Fresh foods, particularly fresh fruits and vegetables are rich sources of potassium. K deficiency may occur due to excess loss of K as in diabetic acidosis, dehydration, prolonged vomiting or diarrhoea. Symptoms of deficiency include weakness, paralysis, etc.

Magnesium

Magnesium is important to more than 300 of the body's enzyme systems. It is involved in bone mineralization, building of protein, muscular contraction, nerve impulse transmission and acts as a catalyst in release of energy. Requirement of magnesium is 350 mg/day. Cereals, pulses and nuts contain 40-200 mg magnesium/ 100g. Green leafy vegetables are good sources of magnesium.

Sulphur

Sulphur is part of some amino acids, vitamin biotin and thiamin. Protein in hair, skin, nails are rich in sulphur. There is no recommended intake and no known deficiency. Protein foods supply plentiful amounts of sulphur.

It is to be noted that minerals actions are co-ordinated e.g. Na, K, Chloride help in maintaining fluid balance; whenever an anion moves, a cation moves. Thus maintains the balance. Na, Cl, K, Ca, Mg help in nerve transmission and muscle contraction and regulate blood pressure. Ca, P and Mg form bones and teeth. Consuming enough of these minerals is not difficult if foods are chosen from each of the 5 food groups.

Trace Minerals

It is now known that a large number of minerals are required in trace amounts. Taken all together, they are only a bit of dust, hardly enough to fill a teaspoon. But they perform a wide range of functions in the body. Some of the trace elements important for human nutrition are zinc, iron, copper, selenium, cobalt, fluoride, manganese, chromium, iodine, molybdenum, arsenic, nickel, vanadium, silicon etc. Essentiality of some of these trace elements for humans are well-established but our understanding of many trace minerals is just starting to emerge. The role of the important ones has been discussed below:

Iron

Total iron content of an adult man is estimated to be 4-5 g. 80 per cent of body's iron is present in the form of hemoglobin—a protein present in red blood cells and helps in transporting oxygen from lungs to tissues throughout the body. It is also present in muscles in the form of myoglobin (the oxygen holding protein of the muscle cells).

Role of Iron

As part of hemoglobin it helps in supplying oxygen to each and every cell of the body. Iron also acts as a cofactor (A mineral that works with an enzyme to facilitate a chemical reaction) to enzymes involved in making amino acids, hormones, neurotransmitters. Iron is necessary for the utilization of energy.

Iron Requirement

For adult man and woman, iron requirement is 28 and 30 mg/

day respectively. Iron requirement during adolescence increases considerably e.g: For boys in the age group of 13-15 it is 41, in the age group of 16-18 years is 50 mg/day.

Sources

Rich sources of iron are cereals, millets, pulses, green leafy vegetables, jaggery. Of the cereal grains and millets bajra and ragi are very good sources of iron. Meat, fish and egg are important sources in all advanced countries. Milk is a poor source of iron. Inclusion of about 50g green leafy vegetables daily can meet a fair proportion of iron.

Absorption of Iron

Only a small amount of iron present in the food is absorbed by the body. Diets differ very widely in the bioavailability of iron. Absorption may be as low as 2 per cent to as high as 35 per cent. Only about 2-5 per cent of iron is absorbed from a predominantly cereal-based diet whereas 10-20 per cent iron is absorbed from diets containing meat and fish. The absorption of iron not only depends upon the quantity of iron present in a food item but also on the type of iron present in a food and other foods.

Factors that Increase Iron Absorption

1. *Type of Iron:* Iron occurs in 2 forms in foods—heme iron and non-heme iron. Heme is the iron holding part of the hemoglobin and myoglobin proteins. About 40 per cent of the iron in meat, fish and poultry is bound into heme. The other 60 per cent is non-heme iron. All the iron in foods derived from plants is non-heme iron. Heme iron is absorbed at a relatively constant rate of about 23 per cent. The rates of absorption of non-heme iron are lower, ranging from 2 to 20 per cent and are influenced by dietary factors and body iron stores.
2. *Vitamin C:* It enhances absorption of non-heme iron.
3. *MFP factor:* Meat, fish and poultry not only contain heme iron but also a factor (MFP factor) that promotes the absorption of non-heme iron from other foods eaten with them.

4. Citric acid and lactic acid from food.
5. Sugars.

Factors that reduce iron absorption:

1. Phytates and fibers in the whole grain cereals and nuts.
2. Calcium and phosphorus in milk.
3. Tannic acid and other poly phenols. Tannic acid is present in tea, coffee, nuts and some fruits and vegetables.

In general, the bioavailability of iron in meat, fish and poultry is high. In grains and legumes, intermediate and in most vegetables, especially those high in oxalate it is low.

Iron Deficiency

When body's iron stores start diminishing the person starts suffering from iron deficiency. The severe depletion of iron stores that results in low hemoglobin concentration is known as anemia. The red blood cells in a person with iron deficiency anemia are pale and small. They cannot carry enough oxygen from the lungs to the tissues, so energy metabolism in the cell falters. The result is fatigue, weakness, headache, apathy, pallor and poor resistance to cold temperatures. Since hemoglobin is the bright red pigment of the blood, the skin becomes noticeably pale. Although diet rich in iron may be able to meet daily iron requirement and prevent iron deficiency, that may not be effective in correcting iron deficiency anemia. Iron tablets can be useful for such patients.

Iodine

Iodine is an integral part of two hormones released by the thyroid gland that regulate body temperature, metabolic rate, reproduction, growth, the making of blood cells, nerve and muscle function and moreover these hormones control the rate at which the cells use oxygen, i.e., they control the rate at which energy is released during metabolism. In short iodine is a component of hormones which help to regulate growth, development and metabolic rate.

Iodine Requirement

Daily iodine requirement is 100-150 micro gram.

Iodine Sources

The ocean is the major source of iodine–seafoods, water etc. Plants grown in iodine rich soil also contain iodine. Iodized salt containing at least 15 micro gram/day could easily meet the daily requirement (consuming 10g of this salt daily meets the requirement).

Iodine Deficiency

Iodine deficiency disorders are widespread in many parts of the world. Over 120-150 million people in the world are estimated to suffer from iodine deficiency. It is characterized by swelling of thyroid gland in the neck. Iodine deficiency during fetal stage may lead to mental retardation and in later in life retardation of body growth.

Some foods like cabbage, kal, rape, yellow turnip, brassica seeds called goiterogenic substances, which come in the way of utilization of iodine. In addition there are some geographical areas where iodine content of soil and water and thus locally grown foods lack iodine. People inhabiting these areas are more likely to suffer from iodine deficiency, e.g., sub-Himalayan region in iodine.

Zinc

Zinc is a component of many enzymes and is involved in many metabolic processes. Zinc plays an important role in protein and DNA metabolism in the body and assists in wound healing, bone formation, development of sexual organs and general growth and maintenance of all tissues. It is also important for the taste perception and appetite and is necessary for the storage and release of insulin.

Requirement

Adults 15 mg/day for man and 12 mg/day for woman.

Sources

Wherever protein is present, zinc is also present. So all protein rich foods are good sources of zinc (meat, fish, poultry etc.). Whole grains and legumes, though are good sources of zinc, zinc is not readily available from such sources.

Copper

Copper works with iron to form hemoglobin and is necessary fo transporting iron and releasing it from storage. It also aids ir forming collagen, a protein that gives strength and support tc bones, teeth, muscle, cartilage and blood vessels. Copper is a par of many important enzymes, such as those involved in the nervous system functioning, blood clotting and immune system.

Requirement

A daily intake of 2-3 mg through diet is necessary.

Deficiency

Copper deficiency is rare. It may result in anemia, bone abnormalities

Sources

Organ meats, whole grain bread and cereals, legumes, nuts and dried fruits are rich sources.

Manganese

Manganese participates in a number of reactions as a component of enzymes or as enzyme cofactor. Its deficiency may lead to abnormality in skeletal bone mineralization. It also participates in lipid and carbohydrate metabolism.

It is estimated that about 5 mg/day is necessary for maintaining normal health. Most of our diets can provide this amount. It is widely distributed in many foods, especially whole grains, dried beans, nuts and leafy vegetables.

Selenium

Selenium activates an enzyme that acts like an antioxidant and prevents oxidative damage to tissues much like Vitamin E. Excellent sources include seafood, meat, liver and eggs. Because selenium is found in soil, whole grains may be good source of selenium if the soil is rich in selenium. Requirement is 50-70 micro gram/day.

Fluoride

It is involved the formation of bones and teeth. So helps to make teeth resistant to decay. If fluoride content of water is less than 1 ppm then the person is susceptible to tooth decay. If its concentration is more than 2-3 ppm it leads to fluorosis (discoloration of teeth), nausea, diarrhea, vomiting etc. Fluorosis is an endemic disease in Nalgonda district of Andhra Pradesh and Patiala of Punjab.

Sources

Drinking water with fluoride content between (1-3 ppm) is significant source. Seafood and tea also contain fluoride.

Chromium

Chromium helps to get glucose into the body's cells. A chromium deficiency results in a condition much like diabetes in which the glucose level in the blood is abnormally high. Requirement is around 70 microgram/day and deficiency is rare. Meat, unrefined foods, egg yolk, whole grains, brewer's yeast are rich sources.

Molybdenum

Molybdenum acts as a cofactor in uric acid metabolism.

Requirement is 0.15-0.5 mg/day. Deficiency is not known whereas excess consumption may increase the risk of gout. It is found in legumes, whole grains, nuts and organ meats.

Other Trace Minerals

Other trace elements of significance in human nutrition are cobalt, silicon, arsenic, nickel and vanadium. Cobalt is part of Vitamin B_{12}. Some studies have shown that cobalt is necessary for utilization of iodine. The significance of other trace elements is uncertain.

Conclusion

In this chapter each and every nutrient essential for human health and well-being starting from carbohydrates, proteins, fats, vitamins and minerals has been discussed in detail. It is important to note that the nutrients do not function in isolation. Some nutrients work co-operatively with each other in the body. E.g. Vitamin C helps in absorption of iron. Zinc is needed to activate and transport Vitamin A. Some nutrients are antagonists. Presence of one may hinder the absorption of other, e.g., presence of excessive calcium in the diet adversely effects the absorption of phosphorus. Excessive amounts of phosphates and phytates in the diet interfere with the absorption of magnesium and iron. So the presence or absence of other nutrients influences the actions of nutrients. So the interrelationship among the nutrients finally affects the health of a person. In addition there are non-nutrient factors like colour pigments, flavouring components in the food. It is to be noted that people eat foods and not nutrients. So nutrients are to be treated as a whole rather than individuals.

Dietary Guidelines for Indians

To maintain normal health, one has to consume all nutrients in required amounts and proper proportions. A well-planned diet that meets the nutrient requirements of a person is known as balanced diet. Nutrient requirements vary with age, gender and physical activity.

According to the function they perform in the body, foods are classified into:

1. *Energy giving foods:* Cereals, sugars, millets, oils, fats, nuts.
2. *Body building foods:* Pulses, nuts and milk and milk products, meat, fish and poultry.
3. *Protective foods:* Green leafy vegetables, other vegetables and fruits, eggs, milk and milk products and flesh foods.

Some classify foods into 4 groups:

1. Cereals, millets and pulses.
2. Fruits and vegetables.
3. Milk and milk products, egg, meat, fish.
4. Oils, fats, nuts and oil seeds.

Foods from each of these food groups have to be consumed to get a balanced diet.

The most recent food guidance system developed by nutritionists is the Food Guide Pyramid. It reflects a pattern for

Dietary Guidelines for Indians
Foundation to Nutrition and Health

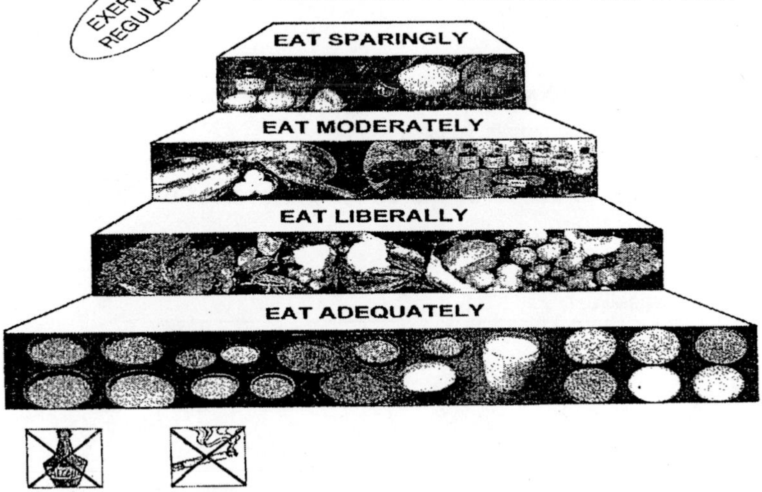

daily food choices. It shows that cereals, pulses, milk and milk products are to be eaten adequately, fruits and vegetables liberally, egg, fish, meat, spice and oil moderately and processed foods, sweets are to be consumed sparingly.

Ref: Dietary Guidelines for Indians—A Manual NIN, Hyderabad, India.

Water—The Elixir of Life

Deny someone food and he/she can survive few days but one cannot survive for even one day without water. Water is in fact the largest component of the body. About 50-60 per cent of the body weight in case of adults and still more in case of children is due to water, e.g., An adult weighing 70 kg has about 50 kg body water.

Inside the body water is not distributed uniformly everywhere. Water content of soft tissues ranges from 70-80 per cent while that of bone is about 20 per cent. Body water is distributed as follows:

Total body water	70 kg
Total water	49 kg

(Contd.)

1.	Intracellular (Inside the cells)	kg
2.	Extra cellular (Outside the tissue cells)	14 kg
	It is further divided into:	
(a)	Water in blood plasma	3 lit
(b)	Interstitial water (water in tissue spaces)	6 lit
(c)	Lymph in the lymphatic vessels	5 lit

Distribution of water in the body is shown in the following diagram:

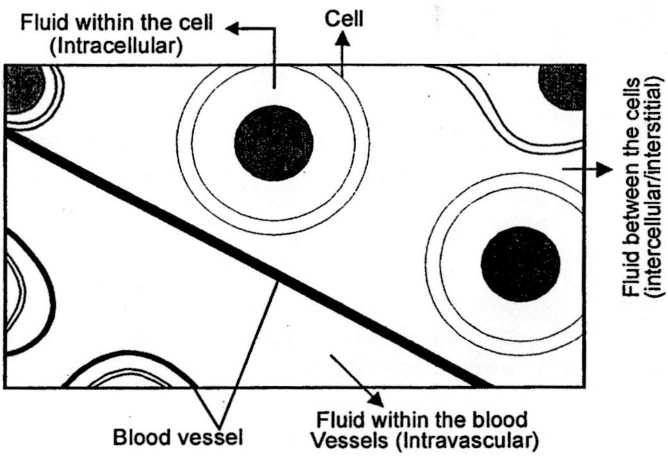

Fig. 3: Distribution of Water in Body

Role of Water in the Body

Water in the body fluids:

1. Carries nutrients and waste products through out the body. It provides nutrients to the cell and helps in elimination of waste from the cells.
2. Actively participates in many chemical reactions.
3. Serves as a solvent for minerals, vitamins, amino acids, glucose and a number of other small molecules.
4. Acts as a lubricant and cushion around eyes, spinal cord.
5. Helps in body temperature regulation.
6. Maintains blood volume.

In the body water is the medium in which all chemical reactions take place. Every cell has a fluid of exact composition, which provides the necessary ingredients to the cell and takes away the end-products of chemical reactions within the cell. These fluids are constantly losing and replacing substances but the composition in each compartment remarkably remains constant. This is known as water balance. Water imbalances can be devastating so the amount of fluid in the body is tightly controlled. The body tries to maintain the water balance as much as possible by adjusting water intake and output. The following Table gives an idea of water intake and water loss per day for an adult weighing 70 kg.

Water Intake	*Temperate Climate (ml)*	*Tropical Climate (ml)*
Drinking water	1500	2000-5000
In food	1000	1300-2000
By oxidation of carbohydrates, fats and proteins in tissues	300	300
Total	**2800**	**3300-7300**
Water loss		
In urine	1500	1000-1500
Via skin (sweating)	800	1800-5200
Via lungs	400	400
In faeces	100	100-200
Total	**2800**	**3300-7300**

Source: Advanced textbook on Food and Nutrition, Dr. Swaminathan, p. 433.

Water Intake

Thirst and satiety influence water intake, in response to change sensed by the mouth, hypothalamus and nerves. When the blood is too concentrated (having lost water but not dissolved substances), the mouth becomes dry and the person responds by drinking water. When hypothalamus detects that the blood is too concentrated, it also initiates drinking behaviour. Nerves also play a role.

Thirst drives a person to seek water but it lags behind the body's need. A water deficiency that develops slowly can switch on drinking behaviour in time to prevent serious dehydration. But if deficiency develops fast then thirst is not a reliable indicator. Also thirst itself is not a remedy. A person must notice the thirst signal, pay attention and take time to get a drink. Example, the long distance runner, the gardner in hot weather, the child busy playing and elderly person whose thirst sensation is blunted can experience serious dehydration if they rely on thirst as an indicator of need for water.

Dehydration may develop if there is water deprivation or excessive water loss. The symptoms progress rapidly from thirst, to weakness, to exhaustion and delirium and end in death if not corrected. Water is also obtained from foods and beverages. Most fruits and vegetables contain upto 95 per cent water. Water is also generated during metabolism.

Water Loss

The body must excrete a minimum of about 500 ml of water each day as urine—enough to carry the waste products generated by a day's metabolic activities. Above this, the excretion adjusts to balance intake. If a person drinks more water urine becomes more dilute. In addition, water is lost from lungs as vapour and from skin as sweat. Some water is also lost in feces. Water lost from the lungs and skin accounts for almost one half of the daily losses even when a person is not visibly perspiring (insensible water losses).

Water Imbalance

Normally, the body defends itself successfully against fluid and electrolyte balance (water and electrolytes usually move together. Therefore, whenever water lost electrolytes are also lost). However, a person may encounter situations of imbalance, which may be beyond the ability of the body to compensate. Example, in case of heavy sweating, vomiting, diarrhoea, burns, wounds when there may be excess water loss.

Effects of Imbalance

Water depletion leads to change in body fluids. A reduction in volume of the extra cellular fluid and intracellular fluid take place.

Urine output is reduced. There is a rapid decrease in body weight and a state of dehydration of the cells occurs. After a few days, a decrease in plasma volume (and also in blood volume) occurs which will reduce cardiac output and lead to circulatory failure. An adult who has lost 5 to 10 liters of water from the body will be seriously ill and death will occur when the water loss from the body is about 15 liters.

Fluid balance, apart from other factors discussed above, is influenced by physical exercise and environmental stress. That is why an athlete athlete/sports person has to pay special attention to maintain normal fluid balance.

Methods for Measurement of Hydration Status

Body water deficit, if any is to be assessed early so that fluid balance can be restored as soon as possible. For this a number of methods have been developed. The methods for measuring the fluid balance status are classified into:

1. Complex Methods.
2. Simple Methods.

Complex Methods

These methods are actually the 'gold standards' for hydration assessment. There are 2 methods:

1. Total Body Water

Total body water is assessed by measuring the dilution of trace amounts of an isotope (usually deuterium oxide). A known volume and in accordance with fluid intake and fluid loss from other avenues helps in maintaining fluid volume. But it is impractical to measure the exact urine volume on a daily basis. So urine concentration as indicated by urine specific gravity, urine osmolality and urine colour can be used to assess the hydration status.

Since plasma osmolality stimulates regulation of reabsorption by kidney, there is slight delay at this stage. In addition intake of fluids and diet influences the urine concentration. So use of a urine sample from the first void (urination) of the morning following an overnight fast improves the reliability of this method.

2. Body Mass

The difference between pre-and post-exercise body mass give an indication of hydration status. This technique implies that 1g of loss of body mass is equivalent to 1 ml of water loss. The uses of this method are limited by the fact that body mass also changes due to energy imbalance over a long period of time. So body measurement is a useful method for assessment of hydration status for short period of time only.

Other Markers

1. *Blood:* Plasma volume, plasma sodium and fluid balance hormones. These methods are analytically complex, expensive and invasive and they are not influenced by a number of factors. Therefore, they are less useful.
2. *Bioelectrical impedance:* It is based on the principle that current resistance (electrical impedance) varies inversely with tissue water and electrolyte content. It is an easy and rapid method but is influenced by shifts of body concentration of isotope is taken into the body. After this tracer isotope is distributed equally throughout the body fluids, the new concentration of the isotope is determined in a sample of body fluid (blood, saliva etc). Then Total Body Water is calculated, based on the principle that a low concentration of the isotope in the sample means that the body fluid volume must be relatively large and vice versa.

Plasma Osmolality

Exercise sweat losses, if not replaced, reduce body water. So plasma volume and extra cellular water decrease as they provide the fluid for sweat. I other words sweat removes relatively more water from body fluids then solutes like sodium and chloride. So these osmotically active solutes build up in the blood plasma. Thus the increase in plasma osmotic pressure is proportional to the decrease in total body water and plasma osmolality returns to the normal values after rehydration.

These two methods of measurement of hydration status are good for sports science, medicine and for researchers but because they require considerable methodological control, expense and analytical expertise, they are not of practical use for monitoring day-to-day hydration status during training/competition.

Simple Methods

1. Urine Analysis

Urine is a fluid containing water and other substances and the concentration of those substance increases with a reduction in urine volume. Urine output is roughly 1-2 lit/day but can be increased 10fold when large volume of water are consumed. The ability of the body to vary urine volume fluids between intracellular and extracellular compartments during exercise, sweating, rehydration etc. and thus reduce the accuracy of this method.

2. Saliva

The salivary osmolality is influenced by changes in hydration but it is not a reliable marker because of huge individual differences.

3. Clinical Signs and Symptoms

Clinical signs and symptions of dehydration such as dizziness, headache, tachycardia etc. are too general and subjective and therefore are not a reliable indicators.

In a research paper by Samuel N. Cheuvrant, Michal N. Sawka of U.S. Army Research Institute of Environmental Medicine have discussed the hydration assessment index thresholds. Recommended hydration assessment index threshold assessment technique and their practicality and cut off mark have been shown below:

Technique	*Athlete Practicality*	*Cut off*
1. Change in Total Body Water	Low	<2%
2. Plasma osmolality (m Osm)	Medium	<290
3. Urine Specific Gravity (g/ml)	High	<1.020
Urine Osmolality (mOSm)	High	<700
Urine colour	High	<4
Change in body mass	High	<1%

Hydration Assessment of Athletes

WUT is a memory device designed to simplify athlete self-monitoring of day-to-day hydration status. The concept for "WUT" is based on sound scientific principles of hydration assessment, but purposely requires nothing more than a body weight scale. W stands for "weight". Athletes should maintain a day-to-day stable body weight. Day-to-day body weight losses in excess of 1 per cent may be an indication of dehydration e.g. Loss of 0.45 kg for an athlete weighing 45.5 kg may be considered as an indication of dehydration.

U Stands for Urine

It is normal to produce more urine when body water is high and less urine when body water is low. Therefore, urine volume is generally more related to body water or hydration level than to drinking pattern. So if sweat losses are high, less urine may be produced despite normal or even increased intake. Low urine production can cause it to be more concerned and a darker colour. A reduced daily urine frequency and darkening of urine colour in a sample taken during the first urination of the morning may be an indication of dehydration. Combine urine information on thirst or body weight to be more certain.

T Stands for "Thirst"

The absence of thirst does not indicate the absence of dehydration. However, the presence of thirst is an indication of dehydration and the need to drink. Therefore, if thirst is present, combine that with urine or body weight information to be more certain.

Simple Tests to Determine If You Are Dehydrated

There are 3 simple questions one can ask to determine if one is dehydrated.

1. Am I thirsty?
2. Is my morning urine dark yellow?
3. Is my body weight this morning noticeably lower when compared to yesterday morning?

If answer to any one of these questions is "yes" you may be dehydrated. If the answer to any two of these questions is "yes", it is likely that you are dehydrated. If the answer to all three of these questions is "yes", it is very likely that you are dehydrated.

Drinking too little or too much water during exercise can be dangerous to your health and can worsen your performance. Here are some tips to help you stay in fluid balance.To determine how much fluid you lose or gain during training or competition, use a chart like the one below to record nude body weight to the nearest pound before and after your workouts. If you lost more than 1 per cent of your body weight, you drank too little during exercise. If you gained weight, you drank too much. If you regularly lose more than 1 per cent of your body weight try to drink more during and after exercise to keep your weight stable. It can be dangerous to gain weight during exercise by drinking too much water.

Date:

Nude weight yesterday morning

Nude weight this morning

Weight change

Thirsty: Yes/No

Dark yellow urine in morning: Yes/ No

Your Comments:

Reference: Sports Science Exchange 97

Volume 18 (2005) Number 2

Supplement.

Ideal Body Weight

If you ask anybody are you happy with your weight? If the answer is yes, then he/she is a rare individual. In fact majority of the people either want to reduce their weight or gain weight. Although their primary reason is appearance, they also believe that weight is somehow related to physical health, physical activity, performance etc. Athletes to succeed in competitions must often meet stringent weight requirements. If proper professional advice is not available then they may develop eating disorders. Ballot dancers, jockeys, wrestlers, distance runners, gymnasts and others whose body weights are often judged in comparison with an ideal are prone to develop eating disorders. Weightlifters also are interested in reducing their weight as this can give them some edge over others in competition. Before trying to either gain or lose weight, one has to know how much he has to gain or lose. For this one has to know his/her ideal weight.

There is no clear definition of a desirable or ideal body weight. Ideal body weights are taken as the weight for height of insured persons with a long life span. Desirable body weights are weight for height of young adults at their best physical performance. A much simpler and more acceptable measure is the ratio of weight and height. The body mass index is calculated as follows:

$$\text{BMI} = \frac{\text{Weight (kg)}}{\{\text{Height (m)}\}^2}$$

BMI <18.5: Undernourished

18.5-25: Normal

25-30: Over weight

>30: Obese

After knowing one's weight, one has to calculate the difference between his actual weight and his ideal body weight, i.e., if BMI is more than 30, then he has to calculate the weight to be achieved so that his BMI comes to normal. One has to understand that he/she is either overweight or under weight because of wrong foods. Before planning on actual diets one has to keep the following in mind:

1. A progressive weight loss/gain of one to two pounds a week is considered safe.
2. No foods should be forbidden as that only makes them more attractive.

3. Eating 3 meals and one to two snacks each day is crucial to minimize the possibility of getting hungry. People tend to overeat when hungry.
4. Portion control is vital. So measuring and weighing food is important because 'eyeballing' is not always accurate.
5. Variety, balance and moderation are crucial to satisfy all nutrient needs.
6. Weighing is important but should not be done everyday because 1 to 2 pound weight gains and losses can occur on a daily basis due to fluid shifts. Weekly weigh-ins are more accurate and less likely to cause disappointment.

Find a Permanent Solution to Overweight

Just as an artist can mould his statues from clay and bronze so can we mold and remold our bodies with right foods. Any person, whose bone structure is normal, can just have a trim, vital body if he is willing to work for it.

It is a fact that if a person is overweight, it is because he/she has eaten more food than his/her body needs and this excess has been stored as fat. This is true regardless of how little one eats in comparison to a slender, active person. Some people require less food because they take relatively little exercise. So to become slender either eat low calorie foods or increase calorie expenditure by increasing physical activities. So to become slender either eat low calorie foods or increase calorie expenditure by increasing physical activity. Some of the common misconceptions about overweight are:

1. One is overweight because of glandular disturbances. According to scientists hardly 1 per cent people who believe that they are fat because of glandular disturbances actually have anything wrong with their glands.
2. Many people are overweight because they are bored, troubled, or emotionally upset. They indulge in eating foods in the same way alcoholic drinks to forget his difficulties. Such people do not realize that they are eating for this reason. As long as the underlying root cause is not treated, superficial dietary manipulation will not help.

3. Some people overemphasize both the pleasure of eating and the hardship of denial. Their sense of values is faulty. They believe that the pleasure of eating is greater than good health and looks. These people have to realize that they can learn to enjoy eating non-fattening foods as much as the fattening foods.
4. Some blame it on their heredity. Although genetics plays a role in obesity, one should realize that environmental factors also play an important role and these people have also inherited wrong food habits, which can be altered.
5. Many people try few times, fail and become discouraged or perhaps ill and rationalize that staying fat is the best policy. Research has shown that it is possible to build and improve health even when he/she is on a reducing diet.
6. It is not the occasional parties that are responsible for obesity. It is certain types of foods, which one eats day after day, such as bread with every meal, too many desserts or too much candy or cream and sugars in coffee. Unless one is willing to change those daily habits, weight reduction remains temporary at best. Regardless of how many pounds one is going to lose, he/she will gain them back as soon as one begins to eat those high calorie foods. So learning to enjoy low calorie foods only can solve the overweight problem for a lifetime.
7. One has to consume protein rich foods because protein help to keep the body firm and prevent unnecessary wrinkles. Consuming 1-2 eggs daily is beneficial.
8. Vegetables and vegetable juices should make up the greater part of the reducing diet. It is preferable to choose green or yellow coloured vegetables as they are usually rich in vitamins and minerals and since they are bulky, they prevent hunger. The following vegetables which contain very less calories (less than 5% sugar) may be eaten in any quantity.
9. Cabbage, carrots, cauliflower, cucumber, brinjal, lettuce, bhendi/ladies finger/okra, pumpkin, radish, spinach, tomatoes and vegetables juices made from the above.
10. Some foods like corn/maize, potatoes, sweet potatoes,

yams contain more sugar (20% and more) and should be avoided, if possible.

11. Fruits that yield more calories should be eaten in restricted amount.
12. Another food that supplies vitamins but very less calories is powdered brewer's yeast. A teaspoon of yeast stirred into water/juice before meal supplies B vitamins.
13. Avoid high calorie sweets, desserts, fat in all forms, nuts, oil seeds, dry fruits etc.
14. It is to be noted that an intelligent attitude helps in achieving that so-called perfect figure. Nutritionists' advice to keep one getting one thing in mind—Diet does it and it is impossible to fail. Weight reducing programme should be thought of as a health-building programme. Only and only when one learns to enjoy low calorie foods, overweight problems can be solved forever.

Exercise for Weight Reduction

Health care professionals frequently advice people who want to control their body weight and lose fat to engage in low to moderate intensity activities for long time. The reason behind such advise is that people exercising at low to moderate intensity are likely to stick with their exercise programme for longer times and are less likely to injure themselves. Research has shown that people who engage in regular, vigorous physical activities have less body fat than those who engage in moderately intense activities. Fat use may continue at an accelerated rate for sometime after vigorous physical activity has ceased. The conditioned body that is adapted to strenuous and prolonged aerobic activity uses more fat all day long, not just during activity. What actually matters as far as physical activity and weight loss are concerned is the total energy expenditure.

The intensity and type of physical activities best suited for one may not suit others. It is suggested that the *intensity* of any activity chosen should be such that the person is able to breathe fast but not so fast as to incur an oxygen debt. A rule of thumb is that one should be breathing easily enough to talk but not sing. If one can sing, the pace has to be increased. If one has to huff and puff to talk, then he has to slow down.

The type of activity depends upon what he/she want to achieve and also his likes and dislikes. If one is looking for health benefits, such as reducing disease risks and lowering blood cholesterol, then it is recommended to spend at least 30 minutes each day doing some kind of physical activity. If one is interested in losing weight, improving body composition, then it is better to choose an activity that one can sustain for 45 minutes or more at least 3 days a week. It is advised to choose the activity one enjoys. Some people love walking, others prefer to dance or swim etc. To become strong and firm, lifting of weights is considered to be good. It is to be noted that muscle is more metabolically active than body fat, so the more muscle one has, the more energy one will burn.

2

Physical Activity: The Inside View

Physical activity has a direct effect on a person's nutrition and overall health. Irrespective of whether a person is an athlete, a health seeker, a health counsellor, a sportsman, or a weight loss seeker physical activity does play an important role in maintaining health and physical fitness. Fitness in fact refers to the characteristics that enable the body to perform physical activity. These characteristics include flexibility of the joints, strength and endurance of the muscles including the heart muscle and a healthy body composition.

Flexibility refers to the capacity of the joints to move through a full range of motion. The ability to bend and recover without injury. The ability to bend and recover without injury. The ability of muscles to work against resistance is the *muscle strength.* The ability of a muscle to contract repeatedly without becoming exhausted. Body composition refers to the proportions of muscle, bone, fat and other tissue that make up a person's total body weight. Physical activity increases the desirable lean body tissue and eliminates excess body fat. A person who practices a physical activity *adapts* by becoming better able to perform it after each session—more flexible, stronger and more enduring.

Some physical activities do not use oxygen. They are termed as anaerobic activities. It is associated with strength, agility and split second surges of power. The jump of the basketball player, the slam of the tennis serve, the heave of the weightlifter are all examples of anaerobic work. Such high intensity, short duration activities depend mostly on glucose breakdown without oxygen as the chief energy fuel.

Aerobic activities on the other hand involve immediate use of oxygen. Endurance activities of low intensity and long duration depend more on fat to provide energy aerobically. The ability to continue swimming to the shore, to keep on hiking to the top of the mountain or to continue pedaling are examples of aerobic activities.

Nutrition Supports Physical Activity

Nutrition and physical activity go hand in hand. Activity demands carbohydrates and fat as fuel, protein to build and maintain lean tissues, vitamins and minerals to support both energy metabolism and tissue building and water to help distribute the fuels and to dissipate the resulting heat wastes.

The food is made up of complex components like carbohydrates, proteins, fats, vitamins, minerals, water etc. Carbohydrates and fats provide energy. The primary function of protein is to provide for growth, repair and maintenance of damaged tissues. But if adequate amounts of carbohydrates and fats are not consumed, there will be energy deficiency. In this case body uses proteins for energy. Vitamins and minerals help in release of energy by helping in carbohydrate, protein and fat metabolism. When food gets digested, the complex compounds will be broken down into simpler compounds.

Carbohydrates	—	Glucose
Protein	—	Amino acids
Fats	—	Fatty acid and glycerol

Glucose, amino acids and fatty acids are utilized for synthesizing the energy currency of cell ATP (Adenosine triphosphate). ATP is a high-energy compound, to which the energy yielding nutrients—glucose, fatty acids and amino acids can transfer energy. ATP is present in small amounts in all body tissues all the time and it can deliver energy instantaneously.

In muscles, ATP provides the chemical driving force for contraction. When ATP is split its energy is released, and the muscle cells channel some of that energy into mechanical movement and most of it into heat—heat the exerciser can feel building up. A tiny but essential pool of ATP is always ready to meet the cell's sudden demands for movement.

Prolonged activity involves sustained or repeated muscle contractions that require ongoing use of ATP. This creates a demand. Immediately after the onset of the demand, before muscle ATP pools dwindle, a muscle enzyme begins to break down another high-energy compound, stored in the muscle. This is phosphocreatine (PC, also called creatine phosphate) PC is a high energy compound in muscle cells that acts as a reservoir of energy that can maintain a steady supply of ATP. PC provides energy for short bursts of activity.

During activity: PC → ATP+ Creatine
During rest: ATP+ Creatine → PC

Supplies of PC in a muscle last for only about 20 seconds but can produce enough quick energy without oxygen for 100 m dash. During activity, PC is made available from creatine, a compound commonly found in muscles, with a phosphate group attached. It can split anaerobically to release phosphate and replenish ATP supplies. When activity ceases and the muscles are resting ATP combines to form PC.

Fuels for Physical Activity

Body uses a mixture of fuels. Fuel is not an all or none process. One fuel may predominate at a given time but the others will still be active. How much of which fuels they use during physical activity depends upon:

1. Fuels available from the diet.
2. Intensity and duration of the activity.
3. Training.

During rest, the body derives slightly more than half of its ATP from fatty acids and most of the rest from carbohydrate along with a small percentage from amino acids.

During physical activity, the body adjusts its mixture of fuels. Body makes use of 3 energy-yielding nutrients:

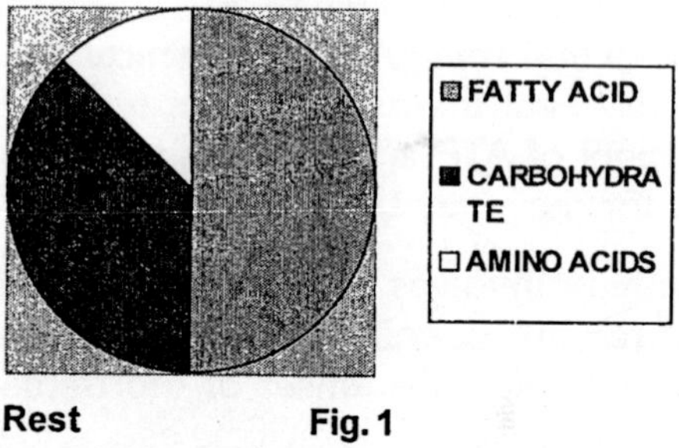

Fig. 1

1. Carbohydrate.
2. Proteins.
3. Fat.

Intensity of the activity and duration decide the type of fuel use. The following Table gives the details:

Intensity of activity	*Duration*	*Preferred fuel source*	*Oxygen needed*	*Example for activity*
Extreme	Less than 30 sec	ATP-PC	No	100 yard dash shot put
Very high	30 sec to 3 min	ATP from carbohydrate (Lactic acid)	No	¼ mile at maximal speed
High	3 min to 20 min	ATP from carbohydrate	Yes (aerobic)	Cycling, swimming or running
Moderate	More than 20 min	ATP from fat	Yes (aerobic)	Hiking

Extremely intense short-term exercisers rely solely on the ATP-PC system. Very high intense activities—the kind that make it difficult "to catch your breath" such as a quarter mile run–use glycogen quickly. Other, less intense activities, such as jogging during which breathing is steady and easy, use glycogen more slowly.

Whenever, a person exercises at a rate that exceeds the capacity of the heart and lungs to supply oxygen to the muscles, aerobic metabolism slows and cannot sufficiently meet energy needs. Instead, the muscles must draw more heavily from glucose, which they can use anaerobically.

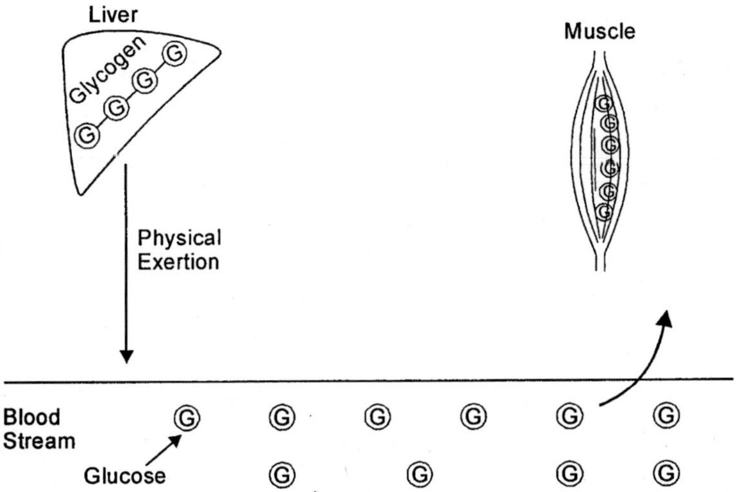

Fig. 2

Glucose

Glucose is stored in the liver and muscles as glycogen (many units of glucose join together to form glycogen). During exertion, the liver releases glycogen from its store in the form of glucose into the blood stream. Muscles use, both this glucose (released by liver) and their own private glycogen stores to fuel their work.

The body constantly uses and replenishes its glycogen. How much carbohydrate a person eats influences how much glycogen is stored. The more the stores, the longer the stores will last during physical activity. Thus dietary carbohydrate bears a direct influence on performance. When glycogen is depleted, the muscles become fatigued. A classic study by M. Hargreaves has compared fuel use during activity among 3 groups of runners on different diets. For several days before testing, one group consumed a normal mixed diet; a second group consumed a no-carbohydrate diet. The maximum endurance time with these diets is shown below:

Fat Protein Diet	57 min
Normal Mixed Diet	114 min
High Carbohydrate Diet	167 min

It shows that the high carbohydrate diet allowed the runners to keep going longer before exhaustion. High carbohydrate diet enhances endurance by enlarging glycogen stores.

As discussed earlier, the intensity of the activity affects the fuel use. Glucose can be broken down completely into CO_2 and water if adequate oxygen is available.

Glucose to Energy: Glucose is a 6-carbon molecule that is broken down step by step to release energy as shown below:

Glucose-to-Energy Pathway

Through these processes, energy from glucose is made available to do the cells' work. Ultimately, glucose is completely disassembled to single-carbon fragments, and the fragments are combined with oxygen to form carbon dioxide. Much of the energy released is trapped and stored in ATP. Details of the TCA cycle and the electron transport chain are shown later and in Appendix C.

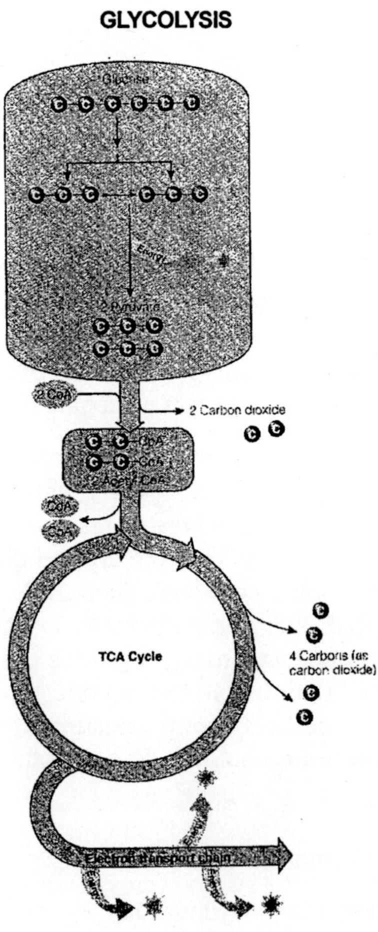

Fig. 3

When the rate of activity exceeds the ability of the body to provide oxygen, the pyruate molecules are converted to lactic acid.

In Absence of Oxygen

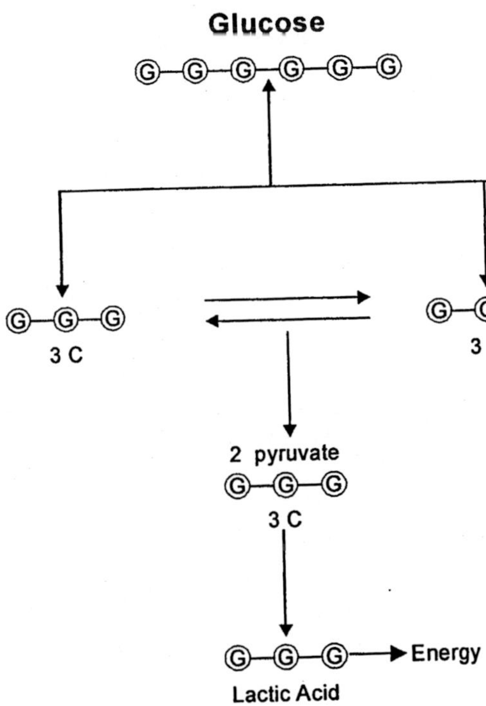

Fig. 4

Lactic acid can produce ATP during intense activity for only 1-3 minutes (as in a 400 to 800 m race or a boxing match) Lactic acid production increases with intensity of activity. At low intensities, lactic acid is readily cleared from the blood, but at higher intensities, lactic acid accumulates, exhaustion sets in and the exerciser cannot continue.

Duration of activity affects the glycogen use. Within the first 20 min or so of moderate activity, a person uses mostly glycogen for fuel—about 1/5 of the available glycogen. After 20 minutes, a person who continues exercising moderately (mostly aerobically) begins to use less and less glycogen and more and more of fat for fuel. Still glycogen use continues and if the activity lasts long enough, muscle and liver glycogen stores will be depleted. After this, physical activity can continue only for a short period. When depletion hits, it brings nervous system function to a near halt, making continued exertion almost impossible. Marathon runners refer to this point almost point of glucose exhaustion as 'hitting the wall'. To avoid this endurance athletes try to maintain their blood glucose for as long as they can. To maximize glucose supply, endurance athletes have to:

1. Eat carbohydrate rich diet (approximately 8g carbohydrate per kilogram body weight or about 70 per cent of energy intake). Percentage of energy intake also depends on total energy intake. Example:. At high energy intake say 5000 Kcal/day, even a moderate diet of 40 per cent carbohydrate supplies 500g of carbohydrate even for an athlete in heavy training. By comparison, a moderate intake of 2000 Kcal/ day, a high carbohydrate for most people, but not enough for athletes in heavy training.
2. Use sports drinks—Discussed in detail in the next chapter.
3. Train the muscles to store as much as much glycogen as possible.

When it was discovered that there is a direct relation between glycogen stores and endurance performance, athletes naturally wanted to store more and more glycogen. Some used a technique known as *carbohydrate loading, glycogen loading or glycogen supercompensation.* It involves moderate exercise followed by consuming a high-carbohydrate diet that enables muscles to store glycogen beyond their normal capacity.

In the early days, athletes were taught to restrict carbohydrates and exercise heavily to empty their muscles of glycogen. About a week before the event, cut back on exercise and then switch abruptly to an extremely high carbohydrate diet a few days before the event. Muscle glycogen increases to as high as 3-4 times the normal amount. But this has side effects that outweigh any performance advantage, including abnormal heart beat, hypoglycemic ketosis, nausea, dizziness and fatigue.

There is another method, which is considered to be safe. Ideally, the athlete in training eats a high carbohydrate diet. During the first 4 days of the week before competition, the athlete trains moderately hard (1-2 hours per day) and eats a diet that is moderate in carbohydrate. During the 3 days before competition, the athlete gradually cuts back on activity and eats a very high carbohydrate diet. This is considered to be effective and does not require severe carbohydrate restriction. Glycogen loading is beneficial to athletes exercising for 90 min or longer.

Training

Training effects how much glycogen muscles will store. Muscle cells that repeatedly deplete their glycogen through hard work adapt to store greater amounts of glycogen to support that work. Conditional muscles depend more on fat for energy, so that glycogen break down occurs more slowly in trained than in untrained individuals at a given work intensity. A person attempting an activity for the first time uses much more glucose than an athlete who is trained to perform it. Oxygen delivery to muscles by the heart and lungs plays a role in this and also trained muscles are better equipped to use the oxygen because their cells contain more mitochondria (Mitochondria are structures present in every cell which produce ATP. They are known as powerhouse of the cell). Untrained muscles depend more heavily on aerobic glucose break down, even when physical activity is moderate.

To make glycogen, in addition to carbohydrate muscles also need rest. So varying daily exercise routines to work different muscles on different days is beneficial.

Use of Fat During Physical Activity

Excess fat in the body is stored. This fat stores play an important role during physical activity. Whenever, the body needs to draw from its fat stores, it is released in the form of fatty acids. The areas that have the most fat to spare donate the greatest amounts of fatty acids to the blood. It is to be noted that these may not be the areas that appear most fatty. That is why spot reducing does not work. Muscles do not own the fat that surrounds them. Fat cells release fatty acids into the blood and not into the underlying muscles. Then the blood gives to each muscle the amount of fat it needs.

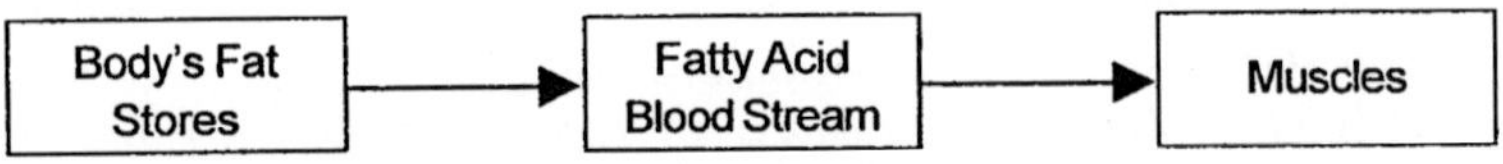

Example: In case of tennis players, one arm works much harder than the other. But fat folds measure the same in both arms, even though the muscles of one arm may be larger than those of the other. A balanced fitness programme that includes strength training, however, will tighten muscles underneath the fat, improving the overall appearance.

Factors that affect fat use are:

1. Duration of physical activity.
2. Intensity.
3. Training.

Duration of Physical Activity

If a physical activity continues for more than 20 minutes, then body starts using its fat stores. Thereafter, sustained, moderate activity uses body fat stores, as its major fuel.

Intensity of Physical Activity

In general, as the intensity increases, fat makes less and less of a contribution to the mix of fuels used. Fat can be broken down in only one way by using oxygen. In fact, the use of fatty acids for energy requires more oxygen than does the use of glucose. So for utilization of fat, abundant availability of oxygen is necessary. If a person is breathing easily during activity, the muscles are getting all the oxygen they need and are able to use more fat in fuel mixture.

Training

It is training—repeated aerobic activity—that produces the adaptations that permit the body to draw heavily on fat for fuel. Training stimulates the muscle cells to manufacture, more and larger mitochondria, heart and lungs become stronger and better able to deliver oxygen to muscles at high activity intensities.

Hormones in the body of a trained person slow glucose release from the liver and speed up fat use instead. Just 20 minutes or more of aerobic activity, 3 or more times each week, stimulates even the untrained body to adapt by packing its cells with more fat metabolizing enzymes and by improving the ability of the heart and lungs to deliver oxygen.

Proteins

Physically active people use protein just as other people do—to build muscle and other lean tissue structures and to some extent to fuel activity. However, protein use during activity and during rest differs.

Muscle Building

Synthesis of body proteins is suppressed during activity and for several hours afterwards. In the hours following this period, protein synthesis increases beyond normal resting levels. Body adapts and builds the molecules, cells and tissues it needs for the next period of activity, i.e., Body tries to remodel part of itself by tearing old structures and making way for new ones. Repeated physical activity, with just a slight overload triggers this process in each muscle cell. This is how body adapts.

Regular physical work of a muscle acts as a signal to the DNA and RNA of that muscle cell to begin producing the kinds of proteins that best support that work, e.g., Jogging. In the first few sessions, the body is not yet equipped to perform aerobic work easily but with each session, the cells genetic material gets the message that an overhaul is needed. In the hours that follow the session the genes send molecular messages to the protein building equipment that tells it what old structures to break down and what new structures to build and within the limits of its genetic potential, it responds. Over a few weeks time, remodelling occurs and jogging becomes easier.

Protein is required for this remodelling. During active muscle building phases of training, an athlete may add between 7 and 28g of body protein to existing muscle mass each day. This increase occurs only during periods of building when the athlete exercises at high intensities.

Protein As Fuel

Muscles speed up their use of amino acids for energy during physical activity, just as they speed up their use of fat and carbohydrate. Proteins at most contribute about 10 per cent of the total fuel, both during activity and rest. How much of protein is used as fuel during activity depends upon:

1. Diet.
2. Intensity and duration of activity.
3. Training.

Diet

If a person does not consume enough energy, in the form of carbohydrates and fats, then body is forced to use protein for energy. In this case, protein, instead of performing its primary functions of growth, repair, maintenance etc., is forced to act as a source of energy. So primary functions protein will be adversely affected. So if a person wants to spare his proteins for its main function, then he has to consume enough carbohydrates and proteins.

Intensity and Duration of Physical Activity

Endurance athletes who train for over an hour a day, engaging in aerobic activity of moderate intensity and long duration, may deplete their glycogen stores by the end of their workouts and may depend on body proteins for energy.

Training

The higher the degree of training, the less protein a person uses during an activity.

Vitamin and Minerals

Vitamins and minerals assist in releasing energy from fuels and in transporting oxygen. This knowledge has led many people to believe, mistakenly, that vitamin and mineral supplements offer athletic advantages to physically active people. But research has shown that vitamin and mineral supplements do not enhance the performance of well-nourished people. Studies also indicate that deficiencies of vitamins and minerals come in the way of sports performance.

3

Importance of Nutrition for Sports Persons

Sports activities demand heavy energy expenditure and therefore the energy requirement of sports persons is comparatively higher than that of non-sports persons. Since the energy cost of each sport activity is different the energy needs of persons engaged in different types of sports activity are also different. Table 1 gives the classification of sports activities by the type of effort and range of probable daily energy requirements in relation to the demands of the activity.

Table–1

Classification of Sports and the Daily Energy Requirements

	Group I	*Group II*	*Group III*
Category	*Power events*	*Non-power events*	*Skilled sports*
	Throwers Sprinters Jumpers Wrestling Weightlifting Judo Rowing (Light weight and Heavy weight)	Hockey Volleyball Kabaddi Swimmers Other Athletics	Archery Yachting
Wt Range (kg)	40-90	60-70	60
Kcal/kg body weight	70	70	50-60
K Calories/day	3600-6000	4500	3600

Source: Narasinga Rao (1996).

Running or jogging for a mile is estimated to expend about 100 Kcal and some runners run 20 miles a day. Cyclists may require about 6000 Kcal/day. It is very difficult to meet such high requirements by conventional means (Garrow and James, 1993). The following Table gives energy expenditure in various types of athletic activities.

Table–2
Energy Expenditure in Various Types of Athletic Activities

Sl. No.	*Activity*	*Calorie Expenditure Per Minute (Kcal)*
1.	Sitting in a chair	1.40
2.	Standing	1.65
3.	Running 7 km/hr	9.0
4.	Running 12 km/hr	20.0
5.	Climbing ladder	8.0-11.0
6.	Cycling (5.5 mph)	4.5
7.	Cycling (9.4 mph)	7.0
8.	Cycling (13.1 mph)	11.1
9.	Canoeing (2.4 mph)	3.0
10.	Canoeing (4.0 mph)	7.0
11.	Horse riding (trot)	8.0
12.	Horse riding (gallop)	10.0
13.	Gymnastic exercises	
	(a) Balancing exercises	2.5
	(b) Abdominal exercises	3.0
	(c) Arms swinging, hopping	6.5
14.	Volleyball	3.5
15.	Bowls	4.4
16.	Golf	5.0
17.	Cricket fielding	3.9

(Contd.)

Sl. No	*Activity*	*Calorie Expenditure Per Minute (Kcal)*
18.	Cricket bowling	5.2
19.	Cricket batting	6.0
20.	Tennis	7.1
21.	Football	8.9
22.	Swimming back stroke	11.0
23.	Swimming back crawl	11.5
24.	Swimming breast stroke	10.0
25.	Playing squash rackets	10.2
26.	Cross country running	10.6
27.	Skiing	9.9-10.8

Source: Passmore, R. and Durnin, J.V.G.A., *Physiol. Rev.*, 35, 801, 1955.

Thus energy requirement is decided by the exercise intensity and duration.

There is a preferential use of nutrients during exercise (Refer chart below). Plasma free fatty acids are the major source of energy during low-intensity exercise (25% VO_2 max) and as intensity

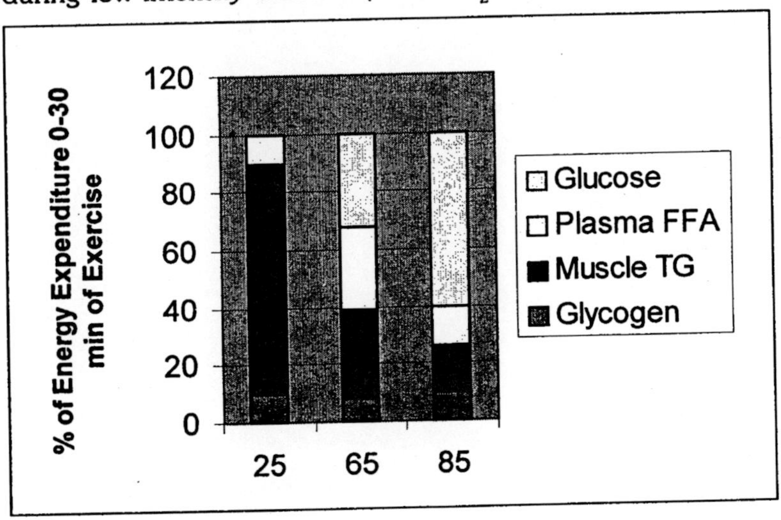

increases the proportion of energy derived from carbohydrate also increases. Therefore, carbohydrate becomes predominant source of energy (Holloszy and Kohrt, 1996).

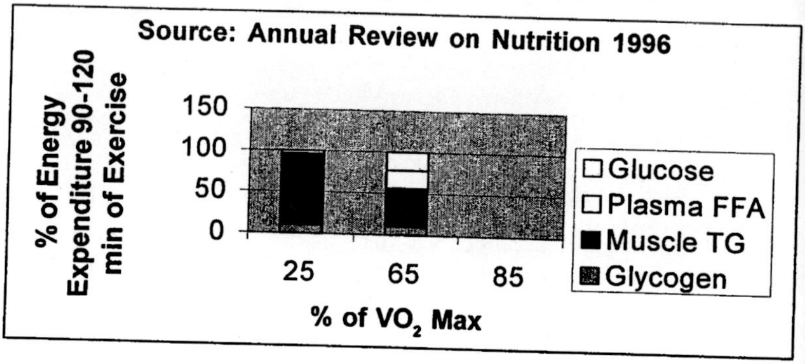

4

Nutrient Requirements for Sports Persons

Calories

Calorie requirements are considerably higher for athletes. Passmore and Durinin (1955) have reviewed the energy requirement for various activities. Depending on the intensity and duration of daily exercise of the athlete, the total daily calorie requirements may range from 3000-5000 Kcal.

Carbohydrates

All carbohydrates are ultimately broken down into glucose. Glucose is the instant source of energy. Excess glucose is stored in the form of glycogen in the liver and muscles and this stored glycogen is reconverted into glucose whenever there is a demand for energy.

Blood glucose is source of energy initially but as the intensity of the exercise increases, energy is derived from glycogen stores. If this also becomes depleted and there is no intake of carbohydrate, the athlete will crash, i.e., he may feel dizzy, light headed and weak. This is due to low blood sugar level. An athlete may also run out of muscle glycogen resulting in fatigue. This is referred to as "hitting the wall."

Athletes require 55-60 per cent of their calories in the form of carbohydrates. Adequate complex carbohydrates should also be provided in the diet. Complex carbohydrates take a longer time to digest and provide a more sustained source of energy. Simple sugars provoke a sharper insulin response, contributing to the dangers of subsequent hypoglycemia. In addition, complex carbohydrates supply needed fiber, vitamins and minerals.

In case of intense exercise, diets low in carbohydrates have proved to be incapable of restoring tissue glycogen levels (Costill D.L.; carbohydrate before, during and after exercise, Fed Proc. 44: 364,1985). Numerous studies have shown poor exercise performance on low-carbohydrate diets. Athletes especially experience fatigue, ketoacidosis (a condition of abnormally high concentration of ketones in the body; a complication of low carbohydrate diets, diabetes mellitus and starvation), dehydration and hypoglycemia (1) Wright, ED: Carbohydrate nutrition and exercise, Clin Nutr 7(1):18,1988. (2) Coyle, E. F. and Coggan, A.R: Effectiveness of carbohydrate feeding in delaying fatigue during prolonged exercise. Sports Med 1(6): 446,1984. 3) Kreider, R. B. and Thompson, W.R.: Ketone bodies and ketosis in exercise, Ann Sports Med 2(4): 170, 1986.

Protein

Most experts recommend 1g protein/kg body weight to meet general needs of the active person. Studies have shown that there is no need to provide extra protein for athletes.

Fat

Dietary fat is necessary, as it is a source of essential fatty acids and for metabolism of fat-soluble vitamins (A, D, E and K). Nutritionists believe that although dietary fat is not necessary, it should not exceed 25-30 per cent of the total daily calorie intake.

Dietary fat is not necessary to maintain body fat stores, since excess calories in the diet will be stored as fat regardless of their dietary source.

Even for an athlete, the need for protein or fat is not significantly greater than for a non-athlete. Carbohydrate is the preferred fuel and critical foodstuff for the active person. These carbohydrates should mainly be complex in the form at an intake that will not only meet increased energy needs but also supply added vitamins and minerals. The following ratio is the approximate dietary composition recommended for support of physical activity.

Carbohydrate: 55 per cent to 60 per cent of total calories.

Protein: 10 per cent to 15 per cent of total calories.

Fat: 30 per cent of total calories.

The recommended dietary allowances for athletes are given below:

Recommended Dietary Allowances for Athletes

Nutrients	*Daily Requirements*
Calories (Kcal)	3000-5000
Protein (g)	60-90
Fat (g)	80-150
Calcium (g)	0.6-0.8
Iron (mg)	20-30
Vitamin A (Retinol) micro g	750-1000
Thiamine (mg)	2.0-3.0
Riboflavin (mg)	2.0-3.2
Nicotinic acid (mg)	26-36
Ascorbic acid (mg)	50-80
Folic acid (micro g)	50-100
Vitamin B_{12} (micro g)	2-4
Vitamin D (I.U.)	400

Source: Advanced Textbook on Food and Nutrition, Volume I, Dr. Swaminathan, p. 607.

Diet for Athletes (g/Caput/Day)

Foodstuffs	*Calories*									
	3000		*3000*		*4000*		*4500*		*5000*	
	Veg	*N Veg*	*Veg*	*N Veg*	*Veg*	*N Veg*	*Veg*	*N Veg*	*Veg*	*N Veg*
Cereals	150	150	175	175	200	200	250	250	300	300
Legumes	50	50	50	50	50	50	50	50	50	50
Nuts	80	70	100	90	120	110	120	110	160	150
Milk	1000	500	1000	500	1000	500	1000	500	1000	500
Cheese	50	—	50	—	50	—	50	—	50	—
Meat fish	—	100	—	100	—	100	—	100	—	100
Eggs	—	50	—	50	—	50	—	50	—	50
Fats oils	—	—	—	—	—	—	—	—	—	—
Butter/ Margarine	20	20	30	30	30	30	40	40	40	40
Vege- table oil	30	30	40	40	60	60	70	70	90	90
Sugar	—	—	—	—	—	—	—	—	—	—
Cane sugar	80	80	100	100	110	110	120	120	140	140
Glucose	80	80	100	100	110	110	120	120	140	140
Vegetables	100	100	100	100	100	100	100	100	100	100
Fruits	200	200	200	200	200	200	200	200	200	200
Fruit juice	1000	1000	1000	1000	1000	1000	1000	1000	1000	1000

Source: Advanced Textbook on Food and Nutrition, Volume I, Dr. Swaminathan, p. 610.

5

Sports and Dietary Supplements

Speed, strength and fitness are the mantra of modern sport. Hitech training methods and relentless sports science research abroad, have resulted in a breed of powerful sports persons. This has led to cut throat competition where milliseconds and millimeters make all the difference. That is why athletes are on a continuous search for dietary supplements and ergogenic aids, which can help them to accomplish more than what is attainable through their own efforts alone.

The search for dietary supplements is as ancient as sports themselves. Early in the 20th century it was apparent that during very heavy exercise, the primary fuel source was carbohydrate (Hortman, 1972). However, there was little applied effort to manipulate carbohydrate intake in the diets of athletes until 1920s, when comparative studies revealed that high-carbohydrate and high-fat diets resulted in increased efficiency of muscular work (Krough and Lindhard, 1920).

Study of the role of carbohydrates in exercise, especially on endurance performance was initiated by Scandinavian researchers in the 1930s (Christensen and Hansen, 1939). The early 1970s saw a craze in carbohydrate loading, when research conducted in Scandinavia demonstrated the effect of dietary carbohydrate manipulation on muscle glycogen and endurance (Bergstrom *et al.*,1967).

The athlete practising Carbohydrate loading or glycogen supercompensation, shifts to a carbohydrate rich diet in an attempt to increase the glycogen stores in his body. The following Table shows the amount of glycogen that can be stored with different diets.

Sl. No.	*Diet*	*Glycogen content (m mol/1.8 kg)*
1.	Carbohydrate poor (1-10 days)	60
2.	Mixed	500
3.	Carbohydrate rich (1-5 days)	900

Source: Narasinga Rao (1996).

But this is no more recommended because muscles become stiff with excess glycogen and athletes may also have trouble adjusting to the diet (Narasinga Rao, 1996).

Diet with high protein content often seems to be the preferred choice of athletes. This probably may be due to more psychological factors and taste than to sound physiology. The fact that muscles are built of protein makes it tempting to conclude that ingestion of excess protein stimulates muscle growth and improves muscle strength. But studies (Darling *et al.*, 1944, Rasch and Pierson, 1962 and Consolazio *et al.*, 1975) have reported little or no difference in endurance performance and strength, when diets of low, normal or high protein content were consumed.

Historically, massive doses of various vitamins have been taken by certain athletes hoping to improve their athletic performance (Williams,1982). The effects of Vitamins C, E and B complex are being extensively investigated for their relative potential for facilitating athletic performance.

Several studies have reported increased mechanical efficiency, physical work capacity, rapid recovery of heart rate after exercise and reduced oxygen consumption after supplementing Vitamin C (Howald and Segessers, 1975). However, Haymes (1983) reported that vitamin supplementation was of no measurable value to athletes' performance. In studies where investigators have created a deficiency in one or more vitamins, there was decrease in performance which could be reversed by supplementing the deficit vitamin (Maurice Jettle *et al.* (1978),Tremblay *et al.* 1984).

Little concern has been shown by the athletes for their mineral status. Costill and Miller (1980) have reported that the electrolyte loss during exercise can be replaced with a normal dietary intake over the subsequent 24-hour period.

Lindsay *et al.* (1988) reported that multivitamin and mineral supplementation was without any measurable ergogenic effect and thus unnecessary in athletes ingesting a normal diet.

6

Dietary Practices of Sports Persons

The dietary practices of sports persons have been discussed under the following heads:

Recommended Dietary Allowances (RDA) and Actual Consumption

The recommended diet for an athlete is high carbohydrate (55-64% calories), low fat (222-31% of calories), adequate protein (12-14% of calories), (Jakovlev, 1975; Malhotra *et al.*, 1972; Satyanarayana, 1985). Studies have observed that athletes' diet is not always balanced, some nutrients fall below RDA and some exceed the RDA. The nutrient, which is often below the RDA, is carbohydrate, which is also sometimes reflected in total calories, whereas vitamin and minerals exceeded the RDA (James *et al.*, 1987; Usha Chandrashekar, 1988, 1989).

Sports persons follow nutritional guidelines based on their own experiences and the myths that have been handed over to them by their coaches have continued to influence their dietary practices.

Harwood (1964) found that most of the advice given by coaches was based on personal experience rather than on established nutritional guidelines. Many coaches emphasize consumption of sizeable amounts of beef in the belief that it replaces muscle protein lost during activity (Cooper, 1966).

Cho and Fryer (1974) reported that most of the physical education students ranked college courses, high school course and coaches as their primary source of nutritional knowledge. Most of these students did not rely on nutritionist, physicians, dietitians, news media, and popular books as a source of nutritional knowledge.

It has been reported that the athletes were eager for nutritional knowledge and advice and were motivated to change eating habits because they believed such a change would be to their advantage in competition (Sarah *et al.,* 1983).

If progress in Indian sports nutrition is analyzed it appears that India has miles to go. Andrew Kokinos, trainer to the Indian Cricketers mentions that Indian players believe that a cup of tea and biscuits were sufficient breakfast on match days. Athletics coach Ken Bosen, visiting Seoul once noted that athletes cafeteria had five separate counters each catering to different disciplines with calories measured exactly. The Indian scenario is quite different. Throwers eat the same food as runners do at SAI centers. In the west, athletes use sports drinks during the events to reintroduce vital supplements, while in India players often drink water from a tap in the field. Comparing Indian sports nutrition situation with that of developed countries is like comparing chalk and butter. Khanna, Bangalore SAI center's sports physiologist admits that we are 15-20 years behind the west (*India Today,* 29th June, 1998).

Energy Bars/Sports Bars

Energy bars, also know as sports bars, are a quick and easy snack for athletes who are often on the go, and provide extra calories for those who are not getting enough. However, it is to be noted that they are not a substitute for whole foods or nutritious meal. The bars can provide energy before a workout, and can help with recovery after a workout or competition.

The recommendation is to eat a bar 1-2 hours before the workout or within a half-hour post workout to enhance recovery. They may even be eaten during intense competition if the athlete can handle the digestion. Remember always stay hydrated by drinking non-caffeinated beverages, too!

The Benefits of Sports Bars

- They provide a more concentrated source of carbohydrate than sports drink and can provide needed energy when consumed during or after exercise.
- They provide an easily chewed and digested form of solid food to help satisfy hunger during prolonged exercise (i.e. road cycling).
- They provide an easily consumed source of carbohydrate and protein for post-exercise recovery.
- They provide a reliable source of protein and micro nutrients for the athlete who is travelling or living in a situation where there is limited access to a range of nutrient-rich foods.

What to Look for in a Sports Bar

- High carbohydrate, moderate protein bars.
- The calorie breakdown should look something like this: 60-70 per cent carbohydrate, 15-20 per cent protein and 15-20 per cent fat.
- Quality protein, like whey or soy, should be used in the bars.
- If eating high protein bars, be sure to eat extra carbohydrates as well.

Beware

- Many of the new "high protein" bars use sugar alcohols to slow the digestion of carbohydrates and cause a great deal of gastrointestinal distress!
- The bars vary greatly in the amount of calories and fat they have. So be sure to look at the label!

So, remember...Sports bars are not designed to be eaten as a general snack or as a replacement of daily meals. Substituting bars for wholesome foods such as cereal, fruit, muffins, sandwiches and low-fat fruit yogurt with sports bars is an expensive option for an athlete and may prevent the athlete from meeting their nutrient needs that are not provided in the sports bar. Therefore, while sports bars can play a specific role in the athlete's sports nutrition plan, they are not intended to provide all dietary goals.

Sports Drinks

Sport Drinks Formulation and Sports Performance

Sports drinks formulation is one of the most researched topics in sports nutrition and this is reflected in its continuously evolving recommendations. Though the appropriate formulation of sports drinks is widely being debated, sports drinks are invading the market in the west and are being advertised by the media. Commercialization of sports nutrition products started with the entry of Gatorade in the market in 1960s. Researchers at the University of Florida, Gainsville were the first to implement the idea of carbohydrate feeding to improve the 'Gators' football team performance (Cade *et al.*, 1972). Gatorade, a mixture of glucose and sucrose in water at approximately 6 per cent concentration ultimately spawned into a multimillion-dollar sports beverage industry. At present there are more than 20 different sports drinks creatively marketed in U.S. and other countries. These products are being utilized by athletes and non-athletes alike and are readily available to the general public. Some sports drinks like All Sport and Sport Toddy, which are fortified with vitamins, are also available, (Elizabeth *et al.*, 1997). The composition of some of the commercial sports drinks is given in Table shown below.

Composition of Commercial Sports Drinks

Product (8 oz)	*Carbohydrate Concentration*	*Carbohydrates*	*Energy*	*Na*	*K*	*Carbohydrate*
	%		*Kcal*	*mg*	*mg*	*g*
Bodyfuel 450	4.5	GP, FR	40	80	20	10
Exceed Fluid Replacement	7.0	GP, FR	70	50	45	17
Gatorade	6.0	SU, GL	50	110	25	14
Sqwincher	6.8	GL, FR	60	55	45	16
Recharge	7.6	FR, GL	50	15	25	13

Na = sodium; K = potassium; GP = glucose polymers; FR = fructose; SU = sucrose; GL = glucose.

Source: Journal of American Dietetics Association, 1991 (91).

Research findings with regard to composition, volume, concentrations etc., have been discussed in detail.

Composition

Sports drinks should obviously contain the substrates preferentially used during exercise. Figure shows the preferential use of different nutrients as source of energy at different intensity and duration of exercise. Since time immemorial glucose is known to provide instant energy, much of the earlier research has focussed on the use of glucose as a supplement fuel.

Carbohydrates

Bergstrom and Hultman (1967) found that glucose infusion slowed muscle glycogen depletion by 24 per cent during a 60-minute bicycle exercise. But, they did not examine the effect of glucose infusion on endurance.

However, contradictory results have been reported when glucose was consumed orally. Influence of glucose ingestion on fuel hormone response during prolonged exercise at 30 per cent VO_2 max was studied by Ahlborg and Felig (1976). They observed that glucose ingestion resulted in a 35 per cent rise in arterial glucose, 60-70 per cent fall in arterial FFA and glycerol and a 2-3 fold rise in arterial insulin compared to the control group.

It was further shown that glucose ingestion is associated with decreased hepatic gluconeogenesis as well as a diminution in lipolysis. As a result hypoglycemia may occur during vigorous exercise following glucose ingestion (Costill *et al.*, 1977).

Bagby *et al.* (1978) investigated the effect of constant infusion of carbohydrate sources like glucose, pyruvate and lactate into exercising rates to know whether these could exert a glycogen-sparing effect on muscle and liver glycogen and found that running time to exhaustion was prolonged by glucose and shortened by lactate or pyruvate infusion.

A study to know the effect of chain length on glucose absorption in healthy subjects was conducted by Wahlqvist *et al.* (1978), using monosaccharides, disaccharides, pentasaccharides and polysaccharides consisting exclusively of glucose. They found no significant difference between the time course of absorption of glucose.

The whole concept of glucose feeding during exercise took a new turn, when Foster *et al.* (1979) observed that the riding time of young men and women on a bicycle ergometer was reduced by 19 per cent when they consumed a 300 ml solution containing 75 g glucose, 30 minutes before exercise compared to the control.

From the above studies it can be inferred that, although glucose is an important metabolic fuel during exercise, it cannot be used as a sole supplement mainly because of its stimulatory influence on insulin. Therefore, investigators have examined the use of alternative energy fuels such as fructose, sucrose etc.

The main interest in fructose stems from the fact that it does not stimulate insulin to the same degree as glucose, it replenishes liver glycogen more rapidly that glucose and increases palatability.

The differential hormonal effect of glucose and fructose has been studied by (Bohannon *et al.*, 1980). They found that after fructose ingestion, the rise in blood glucose and insulin levels were only 20-30 per cent of that observed after glucose load and plasma glucagon levels remained virtually unchanged after fructose feeding.

Koivisto *et al.* (1981) have compared the effect of glucose, fructose and sweet placebo on metabolism during exercise and have shown that glucose ingestion prior to exercise resulted in hypoglycemia, whereas fructose is associated with a modest rise in plasma insulin and does not result in hypoglycemia during exercise.

The effects of feeding fructose or glucose on fed subjects was studied by Levine *et al.* (1983). Three days before the exercise test, subjects were maintained on a carbohydrate rich diet consisting of 70 per cent carbohydrate, 15 per cent lipids and 15 per cent proteins. They found that 20 per cent of the total glycogen content was used with glucose trials, whereas only 9 per cent of the total muscle glycogen was used in fructose trial. The authors therefore suggested that fructose feedings spare muscle glycogen but two independent studies by Koivisto *et al.* (1985) and Hargreaves *et al.* (1987) do not support this concept as their study could not show that fructose was any better than glucose, in sparing muscle glycogen.

Studies have been conducted to know the effect of fructose feeding on liver glycogen. Sonne and Galbo (1986) demonstrated in rats that fructose feedings increase glycogen storage by the liver and that fructose fed rats mobilize glucose more rapidly from the liver during exercise.

The advantageous effect of fructose feeding on sports performance has been reported by a number of researchers. Okano *et al.* (1988) have investigated the effect of pre-exercise fructose ingestion on fed subjects during 2-3 hours of cycling exercise and found that pre-exercising ingestion of 85g fructose in 500 ml water significantly delayed the time to exhaustion and the performance was significantly improved after fructose consumption. Instead of fructose, a combination of glucose polymer (85%) and sucrose (15%) was given to the fed subjects throughout the exercise @ 1g/kg body weight at 10 min and 0.6 g/kg every 30 minutes, and the subjects could perform 19 per cent more work before fatigue, thereby delaying fatigue by nearly 30 min (Coggan and Coyle, 1988).

The work of Brouns *et al.* (1989) has shown that fructose combined with other carbohydrates is more effective in prolonging activity in ultra endurance events.

But all is not well with fructose feeding too. Complaints of abdominal discomfort and other symptoms generally associated with malabsorption have been observed during exercise following fructose consumption even with doses that are well absorbed by most subjects in resting conditions, suggesting that exercise might have an adverse effect on intestinal absorption of fructose (Murray *et al.*, 1989).

A study was undertaken to evaluate the impact of exercise on intestinal absorption of pure fructose, pure glucose and a mixture of glucose and fructose (70% F + 30% G, 95% F + 5% G). The results showed that intestinal capacity for absorption of fructose is readily saturated after ingestion of amounts as small as 50g and that exercise reduces the intestinal transit time, can cause incomplete absorption of fructose (Fujisawa, Takuji *et al.*, 1993). This observation has been supported by Adopo *et al.* (1994) who concluded from their study that glucose and fructose in equal amounts has some advantage when taken together by virtue of increase in total exogenous oxidation.

The concept of feeding a combination of sugars has been further strengthened by Shi *et al.* (1995), who opined that use of a number of different carbohydrates, including free glucose, sucrose, maltodextrin is more beneficial than only one form of carbohydrate. Limiting the osmolality and providing a number of transportable solutes, may maximize the rate of sugar and water absorption in the small intestine. In addition, this has taste implications, which may influence the amount consumed.

Medium Chain Triglycerides (MCT)

MCTs have a smaller molecular size, a lower melting point and are rapidly absorbed and enter the liver directly through the portal vein. With the hypothesis that MCT can serve as additional fuel for working muscles, a number of scientists have studied the use of MCT as supplements.

Vukovich *et al.* (1993) have suggested that ingestion of sufficient amount of MCTs may elevate plasma fatty acid concentration, spare muscle glycogen and improve performance.

Contradictory results have been reported by Asker *et al.* (1998). They tested the effect of MCT ingestion on cycling performance and found that MCT has a negative effect on performance (17-18% lower than placebo) and was also associated with increased intestinal cramping.

Concentration

There is considerable debate on the relative abilities of various beverages to be absorbed into the body fluids during exercise. In mid-1970s to early 1980s it was commonly held that solution containing > 2.5 per cent carbohydrate may reduce gastric emptying following a single feeding (Costill and Saltin, 1974). But since then, there is a major change in this view. Early studies recommending ingestion of solutions containing <2.5 per cent carbohydrates were based on the amount of 400 ml test solution emptied in 15 min at rest.

Lamb and Brodowicz (1986) concluded that solutions containing 6-10 per cent carbohydrates, regardless of type are preferable to ordinary water as they minimize disturbance in thermal or circulatory function as well as maintain blood glucose concentration.

This view was further strengthened by Mitchell *et al.* (1989) who showed that by changing the protocol (drinking 150-200 ml every 10-15 minutes during exercise) larger volumes could be emptied despite carbohydrate concentration of 6-10 g/100 ml. He believed that greater gastric emptying was due to intragastric pressure.

The effect of sports drinks of different concentration on sports performance (Moderates intensity) was studied by Murray *et al.* (1989). The different levels of carbohydrates concentration of beverages were 6 per cent, 8 per cent and 10 per cent. It was observed that those drinking 6 per cent solution had significantly improved performance time when compared to those drinking placebo, 10 per cent or 8 per cent solution.

The fluid replenishing capacity of the sports drinks has been studied by Davis *et al.* (1990). They concluded that fluids in the drinks containing 8 per cent to 10 per cent carbohydrate were made available for dilution in body fluids at similar rates. They should therefore be similar in replenishing body fluids lost in sweat during exercise.

A study by Gisolfi *et al.* (1992) revealed interesting results that intestinal absorption is independent of the form of carbohydrate upto 6 per cent level. Later studies have shown that a substantial part of carbohydrate ingested during exercise is available for oxidation, but there appears to be an upper limit of about 1g/min, to the rate at which ingested carbohydrate can be oxidized, even when much larger amounts are taken.

Volume

The replenishment of fluid and nutrients during exercise is mainly limited by gastric emptying. Hunt and Spurrell (1951) demonstrated that the rate of gastric emptying increased 3.3 ml/min for every 100 ml increase in gastric content. However, it is to be noted that, gastric emptying is not a function of absolute volume ingested but mainly depends on intragastric pressure (Davenport, 1969).

A series of studies were undertaken to determine the effect of solute volume (200 ml, 400 ml, 600 ml and 800 ml) on the rate of gastric emptying, and it was found that the rate of gastric emptying increased in proportion to the volume ingested with a maximal rate of emptying attained at 600 ml (Costill and Saltin, 1974).

Although large volumes of upto 600 ml empty faster from the stomach than do small portions, runners generally find it uncomfortable to run with a nearly full stomach as this interferes with breathing. Drinking 100-200 ml at 10-15 min interval tends to minimize this effect (Horton and Terjung, 1988).

Temperature

Research has shown that there are several advantages in giving a drink at lower temperature. Shapiro and Stoner (1968) have shown that ingestion of cold water (2.5-9°C) can reduce the gastric temperature by 7-18°C with a recovery period of 5-60 minutes. The above view has been further strengthened by the study conducted by Davenport (1969) who observed that cold drinks tend to leave the stomach more rapidly than do warm solution.

In their study, Constill and Saltin (1974) observed that roughly 50 per cent of test solution at 5°C was emptied from the stomach in 15 min following ingestion, while only 27 per cent was emptied when solution was administered at 35°C.

Calorie Density

There is a relation between the calorie density and the rate of gastric emptying. McHugh and Moran (1979) concluded from their studies that, stomach slowed its emptying rate as caloric concentration of drink increased with the result that calories were delivered to the duodenum at a constant rate in monkeys regardless, within limits, of the concentration, osmolality or volume of the intragastric meal.

Brener William *et al.* (1983) showed that glucose assumed a slow and calorie constant emptying pattern, soon after filling the stomach, such that 2.13 Kcal of glucose were delivered per minute to the duodenum for 3 different concentrations of 0.05, 0.125 and 0.25 g/ml of glucose solution.

Osmolality

Hunt and Spurrell (1951) demonstrated that addition of small amounts of glucose to water had an inhibitory effect on the rate of gastric emptying. However, Costill and Saltin (1974) showed that osmotic effect of glucose was only effective in delaying gastric emptying when concentrations exceeded 139 mM. Ingestion of hypertonic glucose (278 mM) solution induced a marked delay in gastric emptying and they illustrated that small amounts of even the most hypertonic solutions leave the stomach during first 20 minutes after ingestion.

It can be said that there is enough evidence to show that sports drinks have a positive influence on sports performance. A study conducted by Vaijayanthi Kanabur and Kamini Devi on Indian volleyball players has shown that sports drinks prepared out of mango improved sports performance significantly. The same study has also shown that consumption of honey delays the onset of fatigue.

The commercial products advertised as instant source of energy, when prepared using milk and sugar according to manufacturers instructions provide about 380 Kcal/250 ml. Studies have shown that regardless of concentration, only about 2.13 K cal/min can be delivered. Therefore, none of these commercial drinks can be used as sports drinks just before or during exercise, as there is a relation between calorie density and rate of gastric emptying during exercise.

Ergogenic Aids

In today's world of neck-to-neck competition, a sports person cannot afford to take chance in any area, as minute fractions of time can deprive him of fame and fortune. Development in sports science research and with the advent of hi-tech training methods, the dividing line between the winner and loser is becoming thinner and thinner day-by-day. It is the milliseconds and millimeters that make or mar the records. Thus sportsmen strive to embrace any possible means promising to improve their performance and leave no stone unturned in getting, the extra edge over their counterparts. In this direction ergogenic aids are believed to be essential contributors to success.

Ergogenic aids are reputed to enhance performance above the level anticipated under normal conditions. Virtually, every food at sometime or the other has been promoted as an ergogenic aid. The most popular ergogenic aids include bee pollen, brewer's yeast, wheat germ oil, honey, lecithin, amino acids, Vitamins D and E, ascorbic acid and gelatin. Most of these enhancers may provide psychological rather than proven physiological benefits (ADA reports, 1987).

Stimulants and Sports Performance

Some studies on the effect of stimulants like alcohol and caffeine on sports performance have been carried out. There is a lot of controversy about the effect of alcohol on athletic performance. Some studies have indicated that alcohol lessens the severity of fatigue (Boge, 1939) restores strength (Jokl, 1968) elicits greater self-confidence (Shepherd, 1972).

Ulmark (1963), Carpenter (1962), Williams (1974) have shown that alcohol has no beneficial effect on sports performance.

Goodman and Gilman (1975) observed that alcohol accelerates fatigue by increasing production of lactate. Study conducted by Hanley (1979) also has indicated that consumption of alcohol has a negative effect as it reduces responsiveness, reaction time and co-ordination.

Ingestion of caffeine was found to improve the work capacity as reported by (Costill *et al.*, 1978) who found that the subjects were able to work for a longer period following the ingestion of caffeine, but Jensen *et al.* (1979) do not support the use of caffeine.

7

Nutritional Deficiency and Sports Performance

Malnutrition

In developing countries like India under nutrition starts from birth itself. Because of extensive maternal under nutrition (under weight, poor weight gain during pregnancy, nutritional anaemia and multiple vitamin deficiencies), about 30 per cent of the infants are born with low birth weights (less than 2.5 kg). According to the surveys conducted by the National Institute of Nutrition, Hyderabad, more than half of Indian children suffer from malnutrition. A large segment of the population (approx 50%) suffers from nutritional anemia. Though the data regarding the prevalence of malnutrition among the sports persons is scanty, it can be concluded that the sports persons also suffer from the above nutritional deficiencies. It is said that if a child undergoes a spell of malnutrition, even once during its life before the age of 7 years; the damage caused on the physical and mental growth can be irreversible. Even if best possible nutrition is provided later in life, the damage cannot be reversed. This is one of the reasons why Indian sports persons are at a disadvantage when compared to their foreign counterparts, particularly in power events.

There is a belief among some sportsmen that non-vegetarian food is a must to maintain good nutritional status. It is true that foods from animal origin contain higher quantity as well as higher quality of protein but this does not mean that vegetarians have to eat meat to meet protein needs. What is needed is an intelligent selection of foods. Vegetarians have to consume pulses like red gram, black gram, peas, cowpea etc. Soya bean is one of the richest sources of proteins. It is called meat without bones. But it cannot be used directly as its seed coat contains anti-nutritional factors. To remove these anti-nutritional factors soya bean has to be soaked in water overnight. It should be boiled for 5 minutes and seed coat has to be removed and then sun dried. After this processing it can be used like any other dhal. It can be incorporated in idli, dosa, snack items like pakodas, vada etc., in place of black gram dhal, or it can be powdered and the soya flour can be incorporated in *chapati*, *roti* etc. Milk and milk products like curd, cheese, ice cream, paneer etc., also provide protein. Some vegetarians do consume egg, which is also a good source of protein. The following case study shows that vegetarian food is in no way inferior to non-vegetarian food.

Case Study

What a thrill to behold this year's Olympics in Atlanta. As I watched the parade of athletes and thought about all the tremendous effort and discipline—not to mention the nutritional needs—that went into their performances. I reflected on Dr. Colin Campbell, you may recall, told about the athletes who ate a plant-based diet and outperformed their meat-eating competitors. Although this study took place at Yale at the turn of the century, I found it ironic that none of this research was available when I took part in the 1924 Olympics as a member of the Yale crew. I would have found it especially interesting because I had been raised on a vegetarian diet.

When I was a child growing up in New Haven, my mother adhered strictly to the advice of Dr. Emmet Holt, the author of The Care and Feeding of children. A Catechism for the use of Mothers and Children's Nurses. This diet did not include any meat, which now consider wise. But it also did not include a lot of other things such as raw vegetables, salads, nuts, berries, bananas, cucumbers, lemonade, cider, and so on, which I now feel would have been valuable.

As peculiar and dull as this diet was, something about it must have worked: all six of us Spock kids developed robust constitutions and grew taller than average. Eventually, I surpassed my fathers height by five inches, reaching six feet four, and all of my sisters grew to be taller than my mother. In college, I first went out for high jumping but then signed up for crew in my sophomore year. Two years later, I proudly, rowed on the victorious Yale Olympic crew in France. By this time, I had left Dr. Holt's food regime far behind and ate virtually anything and everything I could sink my teeth into.

We thought, after eating our first breakfast at the Olympic Village consisting of a dry orange the size of a quarter, a roll and coffee-in contrast to our usual fruit, cereal, eggs, bacon, stacks of toast, and milk—that we couldn't win on such a diet. The Yale Graduate Rowing Committee, which contained several millionnaires, came to our rescue by supplying funds to move to the handsome old city of St. Germain-en-laye outside Paris. There we lived next to a castle with a moat and a forest, and took our meals at a distinguished restaurant, Francois, Premier.

As you might imagine, we were served plenty of meat-based meals in the best French style. Back then, most of us had no clue high–performance athletes could survive without meat. Opinion held that if you didn't eat meat at least once a day, you would suffer from protein deficiency.

Only recently have less Olympic athletes started placing a serious emphasis on nutrition. This year, at the largest Olympic Games in history, the game hosts were faced with monumental task of feeding 10,000 athletes and their coaches for 33 days. This meant providing good tasting, high calorie, high-carbohydrate and low-fat meals; more athletes than ever before opted for the vegetarian entrees.

Fortunately, today we have the information as well as the testimonials of many athletes to substantiate the benefits of plant-based diets. Dave Scott, considered to be the world's greatest triathlete, holds a degree in exercise physiology. In his own words, it's a "ridiculous fallacy" to think that athletes need animal protein. He is joined in his views by such Olympians as Edwin Moses, the gold medallist who went eight years without losing in the 400 m hurdle competition, and Muraray Rose who, at age 17, won three gold medals in the Olympic swim competition. Rose has been a vegetarian since he was two.

This year, I was glad to see Olympic champion Carl Lewis crown his career with his best long jump in two years to win a record tying ninth gold medal. Lewis, of course, is a long time vegetarian whose dietary changes developed out of his moral and religious convictions. Several years ago, Leroy Burrell and Carl Lewis traded titles back and forth when they were being hailed as the fastest sprinters in the world—both were vegetarians.

Whether you are a world-class athlete, a weekend athlete, or simply a recreational exerciser, we now know that you can meet your performance objectives, and improves your health by consuming a plant-based diet that meets your energy needs. Even at my present age, 93, I found that switching to a plant based diet improved my health dramatically.

Source: Nutrition Advocate.com

to Champion Awareness of Nutrition and Health

SEARCH: Vol. 3, No 9- September 2005

Breakfast of Olympic Champions

By Dr. Benjamin Spock, M.D.

(Downloaded from internet).

The Female Athlete Triad

Many young female athletes restrict energy intake to improve performance or to enhance aesthetic appeal of their performance or to meet the weight guidelines of their specific sports. This can develop into a potentially fatal triad of medical problems.

Iron Deficiency

Iron deficiency anaemia dramatically impairs physical performance because the hemoglobin in the red blood cells is indispensable for delivering oxygen for the energy processes. Without oxygen energy cannot be obtained and the person feels tired easily.

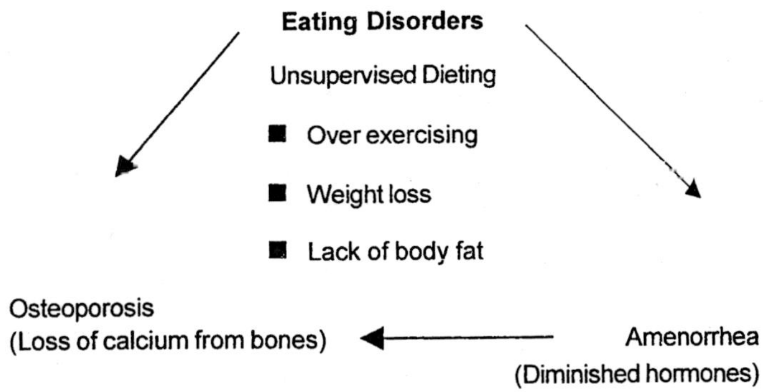

Possible causes of sports anemia are: 1. Lack of iron in the food, 2. Decreased absorption, and 3. Increased iron loss.

Women athletes tend to be more susceptible due to menstrual loss.

Sports anaemia is a transient condition of low hemoglobin in the blood, associated with the early stages of sports training or other strenuous activity. Most researchers view sports anaemia as an adaptive, temporary response to endurance training. Iron deficiency anaemia requires iron supplementation but sports anaemia does not respond to it.

Some suggest that athlete's hemoglobin levels should be higher for optimal performance, however, excessive concentration of hemoglobin leads to increased blood viscosity and a decreased rate of flow. Maintenance of hemoglobin levels at least at the normal levels has been recommended.

Dehydration

About 60 per cent of the energy comes from the breakdown of glucose. In minimal physical exercise this heat production maintains desirable body temperature. But during heavy exercise, heat production exceeds the body's needs and its heat tolerance. Sweating is the main mechanism for dissipating body heat. Endurance events can cause the loss of several liters of water as sweat; unless this is replaced serious consequences can follow.

8

Fighting Fatigue with Diet

Sports is an energy expensive process. A person loses energy and electrolytes during exercise. A sports person tends to feel exhausted after the event. If he does not know how to recharge his batteries it can adversely affect his performance. Boundless energy or freedom from torturing and nagging fatigue is one of the principal factors in helping a sports person to be successful. Fatigue is due to many causes. Every nutrient needed to build health plays some role either directly or indirectly in the production of energy and prevention of fatigue. Therefore, if fatigue is to be avoided, the diet must be complete in every respect.

Vitamin B Complex

One of the most common reasons for fatigue is the lack of B complex vitamins as they play an important role in the metabolism of carbohydrates and release of energy. In experiments in which people have lived on diets adequate in every other respect but deficient in one of the B vitamins, the symptom noticed is fatigue.

To get adequate amounts of these vitamins foods rich in these vitamins have to be chosen. It is said that eating half cup of wheat germ each morning for breakfast and for two weeks taking a heaping tablespoon of yeast stirred into fruit or vegetable juices, milk, or water before each meal and before going to bed has shown good results. Brewers'yeast is to be considered as a food and has to be taken daily throughout life.

Although, some people find yeast unpalatable they notice such a pick up when it is taken, that few give it up after once giving it a fair trial.

Iron

The iron containing pigment (haemoglobin) supplies oxygen to cells. Without sufficient oxygen, energy cannot be produced normally and this results in fatigue. In addition to iron, copper, protein, iodine, calcium, Vitamins A, C, B_6, B_{12}, folic acid, niacin play an important role in building blood.

Consumption of foods such as wheat germ, apricots, blackstrap molasses, liver, green leaves, rice flakes, jaggery or concentrated forms like ferrous mucate have shown beneficial results. It is to be noted that blackstrap molasses, the richest source of both iron and copper and is also rich in calcium and Vitamin B_6. If a person harbours any infection, then regular deworming is a must because infection hinders the absorption of iron.

Vitamin C

Studies have shown that Vitamin C helps to prevent fatigue. In one experiment a large group of soldiers were given 300mg of Vitamin C daily for one month, in addition to that received from ordinary foods. At the end of that time, they were sent on maneuvers with a similar group of men not given the extra vitamin. All the soldiers carried heavy packs, first hiking many miles and later climbing a mountain. The group, which was not given Vitamin C suffered severely from fatigue and their recovery from fatigue was slow. The Vitamin C group experienced almost no fatigue and what little they did feel quickly disappeared. If one wants to be free from fatigue, consumption of at least 200 mg of Vitamin C daily is necessary.

Sodium

Loss of minerals, particularly sodium during hot weather conditions also brings about fatigue. This can be compensated by eating salty foods such as salty peanuts, popcorn, soya beans etc. The practice of eating salt on raw mangoes, tamarind, baby corn, guava, watermelon, grapefruit etc., during hot weather is an excellent one.

Frequency of Eating

Another common cause of fatigue is failure to eat frequently enough. It has been found that people who eat small mid-meals are much freer from fatigue, think more clearly, suffer less from nervousness and are more efficient than those who eat only 3 meals daily.

The mid-meals should consist of fruits, either fresh or dried, fruit or vegetable juice, raw vegetables, yogurt with whole grain crackers or small sandwiches of whole grain breads. The mid-meals should be small and less food should be eaten at regular meals unless a gain in weight is desirable. Mid-meals should be taken at definite times, such as 10 a.m., 3 p.m. or 4 p.m. and before retiring. Foods containing fats and refined sugars should be strictly avoided because they are too satisfying to the appetite. The quickest pickup can be obtained from a mid-meal of bananas (it may be recalled that tennis players consume bananas during break) or whole grain breads or foods containing starch, which will digest slowly and gradually over a period of time. If at any time, a person feels more tired before lunch or dinner than after either meal, then it can be said that he/she may not have eaten frequently to supply food needed to produce sufficient energy.

There are many other factors that interfere with energy production and hence result in fatigue. Example, lack of iodine or Vitamin B_1 allows the heart to beat so slowly that insufficient oxygen reaches the cells and energy cannot be produced efficiently. Lack of iodine may also interfere with energy production. It is to be noted that the metabolism of one nutrient requires the other nutrients in the form of a coenzyme or a cofactor. So deficiency of anyone of the essential nutrients can come in the way of energy production. In short, if daily diet supplies all the nutrients, then energy is produced normally.

Sound Sleep

Missing a night or several hours of sleep can cause torturing fatigue. It adversely affects the work performance the following day. If this continues for a long period the person may resort to sleeping pills. Yet sleep induced by barbiturates or any other drug does not banish fatigue. In fact, the longer the sleeping tablets are used, the more nagging and chronic the fatigue becomes. The continued use of sleeping tablets often results in skin diseases, serious liver damage and ever mounting nervous tension. Accidental over dosage can result in death also. Instead if one follows correct diet and develops the will to relax, there is no need to resort to sleeping tablets. Many foods contribute to the relaxation of muscular and nerve tissue necessary to sound sleep. It is believed that calcium, Vitamin D and Vitamin B_6 play an important role in inducing sound sleep.

Vitamin B_6

It appears that B_6 has a sedative effect upon the nerves. Experiments have shown that B_6 is essential to a normal state of nerve health. It is not found in commonly used foods. It is removed during the refining of grains. So to get adequate amounts of B_6 one has to consume wheat germ, brewers' yeast, blackstrap molasses, liver etc.

Calcium

According to some nutritionists, to obtain sufficient calcium to allow maximum relaxation of nerves every person, regardless of age should consume 1g calcium daily. Since calcium dissolves in acid "soured milk" like curd, butter milk, yogurt containing lactic acid, supply calcium in the form most quickly and completely absorbed into the blood. Cheese, whole or skim milk etc., are other sources of calcium. Calcium is also present in green leafy vegetables but it cannot be easily absorbed into the body, because of presence of oxalic acid. A single teaspoon of blackstrap molasses supplies as much calcium as does a half glass of milk Ragi, a minor millet used as a staple food in southern parts of Karnataka is an excellent source of calcium. Stews, meat soups and all braised meats containing bone should be prepared with a little lemon, sour cream, tomato juice or cooking wine in order that the acid can dissolve calcium from the bone into the gravy/soup. Eskimos obtain their entire calcium supply by eating bones.

If a person is suffering from calcium deficiency over a long period of time, then calcium tablets can be taken. Once the body is brought into positive calcium balance, improvement in the ability to sleep both readily and frequently follows.

Vitamin D

Vitamin D is necessary for absorption and utilization of calcium. With the exception of milk, certain fish, Vitamin D is not found in foods. Sunshine is valuable in forming Vitamin D. Even in tropical countries, people who stay indoors most of the time or wear purdah to completely cover the body may also suffer from vitamin deficiency.

Magnesium

Experiments with animals have shown that those whose diet lacks in magnesium become highly nervous, restless, excitable, apprehensive and sleepless. Such symptoms induce fatigue. Sources of magnesium like brilliantly green leaves such as turnip, spinach can be consumed to overcome the deficiency. The high strung, nervous person should eat daily at least one serving of short cooked greens and a salad of intensely green leaves.

It is to be noted that the person suffering from insomnia may also be suffering from other nutritional deficiencies because deficiencies do not occur singly. So all other nutrients must be supplied to ensure sound sleep.

According to nutritionists if a person wishes to enjoy restful sleep might choose his food as follows:

Breakfast

Fruit or juice; egg or whole grain cereal containing wheat germ; whole-wheat toast; milk or milk drink.

Mid-Morning

2 Calcium tablets; a glass of whole or skim milk or butter milk; or a dish of yogurt flavored with black strap molasses or cinnamon.

Luncheon

Fruit or vegetable salad with cottage cheese: milk, butter milk or yogurt junket; custrad or pudding.

Mid-Afternoon

2 calcium tablets: A heaping tablespoon of brewers' yeast stirred into tomato juice.

Dinner

Fish or fruit cocktail if desired: Meat or meat substitute; 1 or 2 cooked vegetables; salad; milk, butter milk or yogurt; fresh fruit, cheese and whole wheat crackers.

Before Retiring

2 calcium tablets; cheese and whole wheat crackers or small dish yogurt.

Adequate amounts of calcium and Vitamins D and B_6 promote health in many more ways than merely by inducing sound sleep. Just as sleep promotes health, so does health promote sound sleep and both health and sound sleep makes for boundless energy, and makes one forget the tired feeling.

Psychological Problems

A tremendous amount of energy is required when muscles are continuously tensed, ready for immediate action. Only a fraction of that amount is used when the muscles are relaxed. The person who cannot relax and who holds himself tense has all the muscles of his body more or less contracted. He is often tense during the day and also at night when his sleep is fitful and restless. To maintain this tension, food is continuously burnt; lactic acid accumulates more quickly than it can be converted to body starch, hence it acts as an irritant; fatigue results which becomes progressively more severe. Persons suffering from such fatigue are high strung, nervous and probably irritable. The only way to stop such tension and irritability is to learn to relax.

> It has been shown repeatedly that the person, whose diet is inadequate, especially in the vitamins of the B family, worries, becomes depressed, fearful and apprehensive and has foreboding of the impending tragedy. These mental symptoms are not conducive to relaxation. Such a person

keeps his muscles tensed and his mounting fatigue becomes severe. Thus a dietary lack can be the indirect cause of fatigue resulting actually from mental attitudes. On the other hand, fears, frustrations, worries, boredom, and other mental-emotional factors can so upset a person that his appetite fails, his digestion and absorption are interfered with, and dietary deficiencies follow, making a vicious circle; as the diet becomes worse, worries are exaggerated, as worries become more severe, the diet becomes worse. The body-mind cannot be separated, either in function or in nutrition. So it is the mental attitudes and general adjustment to life that become the major factors in fatigue prevention. The more happy and well adjusted the person, the less fatigue he suffers.

Much fatigue can be prevented if a person continuously makes a conscious attempt to relax. Droop occasionally and let down, like a sack of meal. Play that you are a rag doll, without bones or muscles. Unless your duties demand alertness, be lazy, relaxing every muscle in your body. Be thrifty with your energy when it is not needed, then you can be a spendthrift when you want to work or play.

It is to be realized that fatigue can be prevented. It is foolish indeed to tolerate it. It is better to get rid of it once for all. Boundless energy is no longer a secret. It is needless to say that any sportsperson who has boundless energy is bound to succeed.

Source

Anonymous Chapter 11, Goodbye To That Tired Feeling Page Nos.110-119. I am grateful to the author of the book whose name or title of the book or any other details could not be traced.

9

Do's and Don'ts for Better Nutrition

- **Eat breakfast everyday**
  After 10-12 hours overnight fast the energy levels go down. So, it is unfair to expect yourself to perform at peak without refueling with carbohydrate sources. The traditional breakfast choices are appropriate choices for this.
- **Do not starve the muscles of fuel**
  Everyday eat adequate carbohydrates to fuel and refuel the muscles.
- **Try to eat every 3-4 hours**
  This refuels the body with carbohydrate fuel at the rate at which they are being used up.
- **Provide the building blocks of muscle tissue everyday**
  Protein sources like pulses, meat, fish, milk and milk products, egg etc. have to be consumed daily.
- **Food to GRAB on the Go**
  When you are rushing around or looking for something quick to snack on the following foods are useful.
- Cooked cereals with low fat milk, sliced bananas.
- A large glass of juice.
- Wheat preparation like toast.
- Egg omelet with loads of vegetables.

- Sandwiches with Turkey chicken.
- Sandwich with vegetables.
- Choose salads with limited cheese. Choose unbuttered rolls and lean meat that is grilled, broiled, baked, but not fried.
- Opt for low fat cheese.

Top Power Foods

These are energy rich foods, which can be consumed to make up for the high-energy demand.

- *Chapati/roti/parathas/naan* with less fat along with dhal/ potatoes/sprouted pulses.
- *Oatmeal:* Pour it in a bowl. Add hot water, this gives quick burst of energy.
- Traditional Indian breakfast items like parathas with less fat, upma (made out of wheat semolina/suji), idli, dosa with less oil, rice flakes seasoned, snack items like shira (prepared out of fine wheat semolina, milk, sugar and ghee), noodles.
- Potatoes are perhaps the best sources of carbohydrates.
- *Egg:* How do you like them? It does not really matter any way you flip them, boil them, fry them, or scramble them, the truth is that they are loaded with protein but the yolk contains cholesterol. So beware of it.
- *Health drinks:* The so-called health drinks when taken with a glass of milk do provide carbohydrate, protein, along with vitamin and minerals.
- *Chicken:* It is rich in protein. The skin has to be peeled off. It is recommended to consume chicken in baked or grilled but not fried form.
- *Water:* Approximately 8 glass is ideal. (It depends upon the climatic condition, intensity of exercise etc). Body cannot function without water. However too much water is

detrimental as it can flush out minerals and water soluble vitamins.

Star Foods

If there were an all-star foods team these foods would be on it. Here's why:

Banana

The perfect portable snack. They're one of the richest sources of potassium, which may help regulate blood pressure, and are good sources of fiber. Frozen banana chunks make a terrific guilt-free snack. Bananas are also a natural antacid and help keep your muscles from cramping.

1 banana = 105 calories, 0.5g fat, 27g carbohydrate, 1.2g protein, 1mg sodium, 0mg cholesterol, 2.2g fiber, 451mg potassium.

Beef

Truly lean beef is a great source of zinc, high-quality protein and iron. Choose lean cuts such as shank, round, flank, and chuck and trim all excess fat before cooking. Broil or bake meat on a rack, so meat doesn't cook in its fat.

3-oz. lean round steak = 163 calories, 5g fat, 0g carbohydrate, 27g protein, 56mg sodium, 69mg cholesterol, 0g fiber, 13% RDA for iron, 32$ for zinc, 41 per cent for Vitamin B_{12}.

Beans-Legumes

An excellent source of fiber (important for keeping blood sugar and cholesterol levels under control). In fact, beans provide even more soluble fiber than oats. They're high in protein and a good source of folic acid, a B vitamin important for building protein and red blood cells.

1/2 cup serving = 112 calories, 0.4g fat, 21g carbohydrate, 7.5g protein, 1mg sodium, 0mg cholesterol, 7.7g fiber, 304mg potassium, 11 per cent RDA for folic acid.

Broccoli

A wonder food!—one of the best nutritional bets around. Not only is broccoli high in fiber and Vitamin C, it provides folic acid, calcium, magnesium and iron.

1 cup, cooked = 46 calories, 0.4g fat, 9g carbohydrate, 5g protein, 16mg sodium, 0mg cholesterol, 4.8g fiber, 164 per cent RDA for Vitamin C, 42 per cent RDA for Vitamin A, 17 per cent for calcium, 24 per cent for folic acid.

Brown Rice

A good source of complex carbohydrates that provides twice as much fiber as white rice. Moreover, it beats white rice for almost every nutrient, including zinc, magnesium, protein, Vitamin B_6 and selenium.

1/2 cup serving = 116 calories, 0.6g fat, 25g carbohydrate, 2.5g protein, 0mg sodium, 0mg cholesterol, 0.6g fiber.

Carrot Juice

Probably the most concentrated source of beta-carotene, which, in addition to its possible role as a cancer fighter, may play a key role in preventing the formation of cataracts later in life. Beta-carotene, a source of Vitamin A, also may boost your immune system's ability to fight bacterial and viral infections.

1/2 cup serving = 49 calories, 0.2g fat, 11g carbohydrate, 1g protein, 36mg sodium, 0mg cholesterol, 1.2g fiber, about 33 per cent RDA for Vitamin A.

Low Fat or Fat Free Cheeses

Great sources of calcium, but read nutritional labels carefully: Some of these cheeses aren't much lower in fat than their regular counterparts, and they can be high in sodium. Choose one that contains 5 grams or less fat per ounce.

1–oz serving Alpine Lace = 85 calories, 5 g fat, 7g protein, 85mg sodium, 20mg cholesterol, 35 per cent RDA for calcium.

Chicken

Three ounces of skinless chicken breast has only 3 grams of fat and contains Vitamin B_6, a nutrient important for metabolizing protein. Dark meat has more fat than white, but also more B vitamins, iron, zinc and other nutrients. Unlike popular belief, skin fat does not "migrate" into the meat, so cook the chicken with the skin on and remove after cooking. This keeps the chicken moist.

3-oz. Breast, no skin, roasted = 140 calories, 2.9g fat, 0g carbohydrates, 26g protein, 62mg sodium, 0g fiber, 58 per cent RDA for niacin, 25 per cent for Vitamin B_6.

Corn

An often overlooked source of fiber and carbohydrate. Sure, fresh corn tastes best, but frozen or canned alternatives are convenient ways to get additional fiber in your diet. Corn also has almost no fat.

1/2 cup serving = 67 calories, 0.6g fat, 17g carbohydrate, 2.5g protein, 4mg sodium, 1.6g fiber, 17 micrograms folic acid.

Dried Fruit

Because most of the water has been removed, dried fruits are terrific concentrated sources of energy and good sources of iron—a mineral that helps prevent anemia. High in fructose, they also can be intensely sweet, making them great desserts or snacks—and they're fat free.

3-oz serving = 203 calories, 0.4 g fat, 53 g carbohydrate, 3.1 g protein, 8.5 mg sodium, 0 mg cholesterol, 6.8 g fiber, 22 per cent RDA for iron, 123 per cent RDA for vitamin A.

Fig Bars

A favourite among cyclists and runners because they pack a strong carbohydrate punch and are easy to eat during exercise. Much lower in fat than most treats, fig bars also supply a bit of fiber–not a lot, but more than most sweets.

2 bars = 106 calories, 1.9g fat, 21g carbohydrate, 1g protein, 90mg sodium, 0mg cholesterol, 5g fiber.

Grapes

Once thought to provide few significant nutrients, now researchers find that grapes are a good source of boron, a mineral believed to be important in building and maintaining healthy bones.

1/2 cup serving = 29 calories, 0.2g fat, 1mg sodium, 0mg cholesterol, 0.3g fiber.

Kiwi

The odd little fruit in the fuzzy brown wrapper proves that good things can come in small, ugly packages. Each kiwi provides 75mg of Vitamin C and 1.7grams of fiber.

1 kiwi = 46 calories, 0.3g fat, 11g carbohydrate, 0.8g protein, 4mg sodium, 0mg cholesterol, 1.7g fiber, 124 per cent RDA for Vitamin C.

Lentils

Good sources of protein and complex carbohydrates, lentils also deliver a good amount of iron, particularly if you're limiting your intake of red meat. Lentils are easier to prepare than other legumes because you don't have to soak them overnight before cooking. Great on their own, in soups or as an addition to ground meat.

1/2 cup serving = 105 calories, 0g fat, 20g carbohydrate, 8g protein, 30mg sodium, 0 mg cholesterol, 5.2g fiber, 12 per cent RDA for iron, 7 per cent for zinc, 9 per cent for folic acid.

Skim Milk

Skim milk is an excellent low-fat source of calcium and Vitamin D–both important for maintaining healthy bones. Research suggests that you have less risk of developing colon cancer with high blood levels of Vitamin D than with low levels. But don't turn to supplements for Vitamin D: large amounts can be toxic.

8 = oz. = 80 calories, 0.4g fat, 11g carbohydrate, 8g protein, 4mg. cholesterol, 117 mg sodium, 0g fiber, 24 per cent RDA for Vitamin D, 28 per cent for calcium.

Oatmeal

A good source of soluble fiber, and then some: In a research study, adding 2 ounces a day of oatmeal to a low-fat diet significantly lowered subjects' blood cholesterol in about four weeks.

1/2 cup serving = 73 calories, 1.2g fat, 13g carbohydrate, 3g protein, 1 mg sodium, 0mg cholesterol, 2.7g fiber.

Orange Juice

Besides being an excellent source of Vitamin C, one 6-ounce glass provides nearly as much potassium as a banana and about 23 percent of the RDA for the sometimes-hard-to-find B vitamin folic acid.

6 oz. = 76 calories, 0.3g fat, 15g carbohydrate, 1g protein, 1mg sodium, 0.1g fiber, 340mg potassium, 142 per cent RDA for Vitamin C, 23 per cent RDA for folic acid.

Papaya

Papaya is a treasure trove of nutrients. One-half of this exotic fruit provides almost as much potassium as a banana and more than 100 per cent of the RDA for Vitamin C. It's also a good source of cancer-fighting beta-carotene.

1/2 papaya = 59 calories, 0.2g fat, 15g carbohydrate, 1g protein, 4mg sodium, 0mg cholesterol, 12.2g fiber, 395mg potassium, 158 per cent RDA for Vitamin C, about 62 per cent RDA for Vitamin A.

Pasta

Pasta is loaded with complex carbohydrates for long-lasting energy, whether you're an athlete or a couch potato. Enriched pasta also provides iron and the important B vitamins thiamine, niacin and riboflavin.

1/2 cup serving = 77 calories, 0.3g fat, 28g carbohydrate, 5.3g protein, 0mg cholesterol, 1mg sodium, 35 per cent RDA for thiamine, 15 per cent RDA for riboflavin, 15 per cent RDA for niacin, 10 per cent RDA for iron.

Potato

The potato is probably one of the most underrated foods. Besides being a powerhouse of complex carbohydrates, a 6-ouncer also provides almost twice as much potassium as a banana, just over one-third of the RDA for Vitamin C and 66 per cent of the RDA for iron. It's also a good source of copper, which most people tend to be short on.

6-oz. baked, with skin = 337 calories, 0.2g fat, 78g carbohydrate, 7g protein, 35mg sodium, 0mg cholesterol, 4g fiber, 974 g potassium, 38 per cent RDA for Vitamin C, 66 per cent RDA for iron, 70 per cent RDA for copper, 56 per cent RDA for Vitamin B_6.

Salmon

Salmon is one of the richest sources for omega-3 fatty acids, which may provide some protection against heart disease. Eating salmon or other ocean fish like mackerel, herring or tuna twice a week may be enough for you to reap the health benefits. Fish oil may also fight arthritis, alleviate psoriasis and reduce high blood pressure. Salmon is also an excellent source of selenium, which may play a role in cancer prevention.

3-oz. cooked = 45 calories, 0.6g fat, 0g carbohydrate, 0g fiber, 40 micrograms selenium, 42 per cent RDA for niacin, 35 per cent RDA for calcium. Most types of salmon provide about 1g omega-3 fatty acids.

Strawberries

Sweet, delicious strawberries are excellent sources of Vitamin C and fiber. They also contain ellagic acid and beta-carotene, which may prove important in cancer prevention.

1 cup serving = 45 calories, 0.6g fat, 11g carbohydrate, 1g protein, 2mg sodium, 0mg cholesterol, 2.2g fiber, 141 per cent RDA for Vitamin C.

Water

The most critical nutrient in your body, it's needed for just about everything that happens, and you lose it fast: at least 2 cups daily just exhaling; 10 cups through normal waste and body cooling: 1 to 2 quarts per hour running, biking or working out. Eight glasses a day is enough for sedentary people, but if you are physically active, you need more. Drink 8 to 20 ounces of water about 15 minutes before working out. If you run, drink at least 2 cups of water for every pound you lose on your course.

Whole-Grain Cereals

Besides providing lots of complex carbohydrates, they're a great way to get fiber in your diet—a prevention measure that the National Cancer Society strongly recommends. What's more, research suggest that eating a high-fiber cereal at breakfast may curb your appetite at lunch. Read the labels: a cereal should contain at least 5 grams of fiber and no more than 1 or 2 grams of fat per serving.

Fat Free Yogurt

Among the few truly excellent sources of calcium-452 mg per 8 ounce carton—and riboflavin, yogurt's also a strong source of Vitamin B_{12}. Use it to reduce fat in your diet: substitute it for sour cream in casseroles or sauces: mix with herbs for vegetable dip; blend with fruit for a thick drink; stir into soups to make them creamy. Frozen, it's an excellent substitute for ice cream. To cut calories in half in flavored yogurts, choose brands artificially sweetened with NutraSweet.

8 oz. serving, plain = 127 calories, 0.4g fat, 17g carbohydrate, 13g protein, 174mg sodium, 4 mg cholesterol, 0g fiber 45 per cent RDA for calcium; 31 per cent for riboflavin, 23 per cent RDA for vitamin B_{12}.

Information Supplied By

Megan Mangano, UNH B.S. in Nutritional Sciences, SDSU Dietetic Intern Clark, Nancy, MS, RD. Nancy Clark's Sports Nutrition Guidebook, 2nd Edition, 1997. Brookline, MA: Nancy Clark.

Rosenbloom, Christine A., Ph.D, RD, Editor. ADA: Sports Nutrition: A Guide for the Professional Working with Active People, 3rd Edition, 2000. Chicago, Illinois: The American Dietetic Association.

10

Pre-Competition Nutrition

The real winning edge comes from intelligent dietary management just before, during, as well as after the event. Many athletes experience pre-competition nerves, which directly affect their appetite. Stomach cramps and diarrhoea are also common. According to Ms. Nimmi Ittycheria John, a nutritionist, it is wise to keep fiber down and keep with what is tried and tested during training periods.

The following Table gives an idea of the ideal pattern of diet before, during and after the sports event.

	Aims	*Food and Drink Recommendation*	*Example*
The week before	Fill glycogen stores Maintain hydration	Taper training 60-70% carb (7-8) kg/kg body weight low-GI meal monitor fluid intake	Oats/ragi porridge, whole wheat parathas with *channa,* rice with *rajma.* Curds rice with fried fish or *rotis* with *palak paneer,* and orange juice
The night before	To top up muscle glycogen To maintain hydration	High-carb meal (low GI) plenty of fluids moderate-to-low fiber Low fat familiar foods	Pears, apples, oranges and musambi. Pasta (about 3 cups with tomato sauce and 1 tbsp grated cheese

(Contd.)

	Aims	*Food and Drink* Recommendation	*Example*
			or Basamati rice with rajma. A scoop of icecream A small fruit and fruit juice (250ml)
24 hours before	To top up liver/maintain hydration/ keep hunger at bay without causing discomfort. Promote use of carb during exercise	High carb low fat, low protein Easily digestible 500ml of liquid	1 small bowl of wheat flakes/muesli with low fat milk Toast 2 slices of idli with honey
1 hour before	To maintain blood sugar To maintain hydration	1kg carb/kg body wgt. Easy to digest liquid	Sports drink and/or water dried apricots/ dates (8-10) fruits cake 2 small slices
15-30 minutes before	To maintain hydration	125-500 ml fluid	Water or Sports drink or Lime juice with sugar
During events more than 60 minutes	To maintain blood sugar To off set Fluid losses	30-60 g carb/hour High to moderate GI carb 120-250 ml fluids every 10-20 min	Sports Drinks Lime juice with sugar
Between heats and events	Replenish muscle and liver glycogen Replenish fluids	1g/kg body weight carb high GI carb 500 ml fluid immediately after Continue fluids	Puffed rice with sesame and jaggery balls (for children)/Bananas/few dates/Sweet bun
Post-competition glycogen	Replenish muscle and liver Replace fluid	1g/kg body weight carb within 2 hours/ High GI carb	Lime juice/Sports drink Lime rice/ Curd rice Pizza or full traditional Indian meals

Carb: Carbohydrate, GI: Glycemic Index—The ranking of foods based on their immediate effect on blood glucose levels. Those with low GI foods produce slow and sustained increase in blood glucose, e.g., Low fat curd, skim, *rajma, channa*. Those with high GI produce a rapid, dramatic and short-lived elevation of blood glucose. Example, idlis, white bread, corn flakes, potatoes, isotonic sports drink, puffed rice, bananas and raisins.

BEWARE! Banned substances could be there in supplement.

The following ingredients sometimes found in supplements and sports drinks have been either banned by the International Olympic Committee's Medical Commission or have been shown to cause a positive doping outcome in some people.

Ephedrine, pseudoephidrine, strychine, caffeine (if consumed in sufficiently high quantities to produce a urinary caffeine concentration of more than 12 mg/ml). Dehydroepianddrosterone (DHEA), androstenedione, androstenediol and 19 nonandrostenedione, 19 nonandrostenediol and related compounds. Sadly an athlete could fall in the trap if questionable ingredients are added deliberately and not declared.

Creatinine, a popular supplement with Indian coaches and athletes does not feature in the banned list France's Food Safety Agency (AFSSA) experts on Human Nutrition found that increased muscle bulk resulting from creatinine supplementation was largely due to water retention and also concluded that the widespread claims about gains in strength were unfounded. Their conclusion was that the use of creatinine involves a risk disproportionate to its effectiveness. Therefore it is wise to read labels and screen for banned substance well before D day so that the career and reputation of the sports person can be saved.

Source: Mrs. Nimmi Ittycheria John, as reported in Dec 2003, Food and Nutrition World).

- If you will be exercising for more than 60-90 min, choose carbohydrate with a moderate to low glycemic index (Example, Banana, oatmeal, bean soup, apples, lentils etc) Consume 1-4 g of carbohydrate/kg body weight, 1-4 hrs before exercise.

  Consume 30-40g carbohydrate every hour during exercise.

- If you will be exercising for less than an hour simply snack on any tried and true foods that digest easily and comfortably, e.g., bread, pasta. Even an energy bar with fruit/fruit juice with water is also adequate.

- Limit high fat proteins.
- Be cautious with sugary foods like soft drinks, candy, regular soda, fruit juice as they cause a drop in blood sugar level leaving you tired.
- Highly refined carbohydrates e.g. preparations using highly polished rice, maida etc., will cause the same effect. Try to eat them with other nutrient dense foods containing complex carbohydrates e.g. vegetables and fruits.
- Allow adequate time to digest.
- Always eat familiar foods before competition. Don't try anything new.

Refuel After Matches

It takes 20 hours to fully replenish depleted muscle glycogen. As soon as possible rehydrate and choose high carbohydrate foods. 2-3 cups of fluids with a piece of fruit would be appropriate. Getting complex carbohydrate choices within 2 hours of heavy play is important to prevent early onset of fatigue. The traditional dinner would be an excellent choice for post match play. Limit heavy proteins, fats and caffeine at this time because of their diuretic effects.

- Do not avoid protein in your recovery diet. The desirable ratio between carbohydrate and protein is 3:1.
- After a hard work out or competition, your top priority should be replaced your lost nutrients. Remember for every 1 lb. lost, drink 2 cups of fluid. Juices such as watermelon, grape, sports drinks and water.
- Replace electrolytes. When you are exercising you sweat. When you sweat you lose important electrolytes, such as potassium and sodium. A pound of sweat contains about 80-100 mg of potassium. In course of 2-3 hours of very hard exercise you might lose 300-800 mg K and 1800-5600 mg sodium. For this ORS (Oral Rehydration Solution), lemon juice (containing lemon juice, sugar and

salt), orange juice, banana, potato, raisins, sports drinks like All Sport, Powerade, Gatorade etc., which are rich sources of potassium, cheese, bread, orange juice, papads, fryums, pickles etc., which are rich sources of sodium have to be consumed.

- Some sportsmen believe that consuming orange juice with 5 almond powder on empty stomach during morning hours improves immunity.

11
Conclusion

Research in the West has concentrated on few specific areas of sports nutrition namely fluid and electrolyte balance, physiology of thermoregulation, carbohydrate requirements of endurance athletes. Among the many questions that remain unanswered are protein requirements of athletes, carbohydrate requirements of non-endurance athletes etc. Research is going on in areas like sports drink formulation and this is being reflected in its continuously evolving recommendations. In India sports nutrition as such is a green area. Data on dietary habits remains sketchy at best. In a country where malnutrition and anaemia are widespread public health problems more data needs to be generated about the prevalence of these among sports persons as they have a direct bearing on sports performance. In addition every effort should be made to provide 'sports specific', 'tailor made' food for the sportsmen. Since we have limited resources cost effective food supplements have to be developed. Last but not the least, every effort must be made to realize that ignorance is not a bliss as far as sports nutrition is concerned because the gap between winner and loser is becoming thinner and thinner. Success is sweet but its secret is sweat. Putting efforts in right direction is a must for success.

Bibliography

Adopo, E., Perronet F., Massicote D., Brisson, G., Hilaire Marcel, C., 1994: Respective oxidation of exogenous glucose and fructose given in the same drink during exercise, *Journal of Applied Physiology*, 76: 1014-1019.

American Dietetic Association Reports, 1987: Nutrition for physical fitness and athletic performance for adults, *Technical support paper*, 87(7): 934-939.

Asker Jeukendrup, Josephine, Anton, J. M. Wagenmakers, Fred Brouns and Wim H. M. Saris, 1998: Effect of medium chain triacylglycerol and carbohydrate ingestion during exercise on substrate utilization and subsequent cycling performance. *American Journal of Clinical Nutrition*, 67:397-404.

Bergstrom, J., Hermansen, L., Hultman, E. and Saltin B. 1967: Diet, muscle glycogen and physical performance Acta, *Physiol Scand*, 71: 140-150.

Bohannon, N. V., Karam, J.H., Forsham, P.H. 1980: Endocrine responses to sugar ingestion in man, *Journal of American Dietetic Association*, 76: 555-560.

Boge, O. D., 1939: A Study of the means employed to raise the level of performance in sport.

Brouns, F., Saris, W. H. M., Beckers, E. M. 1989: Metabolic changes introduced by sustained exhaustive cycling and diet manipulation International, *Journal of Sports Medicine*, 10: 549-562.

Cade, R., Spooner G., Schlein, E., Pickering, M. and Dean, R. 1972: Effects of fluids, electrolyte, and glucose replacement during exercise on performance, body temperature, rate of sweat loss, and compositional changes of extracellular fluid, *Journal of Sports Medicine Physiology and Fitness*, 12: 150-156.

Carpenter, I., 1962: Effects of alcohol and some psychological processes, *Quarterly General Studies on Alcohol*, 23:274.

Christensen and Hansen, 1939: Respiratorischen qutient und O 2 aufanchme Skandinovsches, *Archiv fur Physiologie* 81: 180-189.

Cooper, D. L., 1966: Nutrition in Athletes, *Journal of American College Health Association* 14 261.

Consolazio, G. F., Johnson, H. L., Nelson, R. A., Dramise, J. G. and Skale, J. H., 1975: Protein metabolism during intensive physical training in the young adult, *American Journal of Clinical Nutrition* 28: 29-35.

Costill, D. L., and Saltin, B., 1974: Factors limiting gastric emptying during rest and exercise, *Journal of Applied Physiology,* 37(5):679-683.

Costill, D. L., 1985: Carbohydrate before, during and after exercise, *Fred Proc* 44: 364.

Costill, D. L., Dalsky, G. P. and Fink, W. J., 1978: Effects of caffeine ingestion on metabolism and exercise performance. *Medicine and Science in Sports and Exercise* 10: 155-158.

Costill, D. L., and Miller, J. M., 1980: Nutrition for endurance sport: carbohydrate and fluid balance. *International Journal of Sports Medicine*, 1:2-14.

Coyle, E. F. and Coggan, A. R.,1984: Effectiveness of Carbohydrate feeding in delaying fatigue during prolonged exercise, *Sports Med* 1(6), 446.

Cho, M. and Fryer, B. A., 1974: Nutritional knowledge of collegiate physical education majors, *Journal of American Dietetic Association*, 65: 30.

Davis , J. M., Mark, William, A., Burgess, Cris, A., Slentz and William Bastoli, 1990: Fluid availability of sports drinks differing in carbohydrate type and concentration, *American Journal of Clinical Nutrition*, 51: 1054-1057.

Darling, R.C., Johnson, R. E., Pitts, G. L., Consolazio, F. C. and Robinson, P. F. 1944: Effects of variations in dietary protein on the physical well being of men doing manual work, *Journal of Nutrition* 28: 273-281.

Davenport, H. W., 1969: *Physiology of the digestive tract.* 2nd edn. Chicago Year Book Medical Publishers.

Dietary, Guidelines for Indians—A manual, 1998: *National Institute of Nutrition Hyderabad: Advanced Textbook on Food and Nutrition*, Vol 1, 1991, M. Swaminathan, Bappco Publication Bangalore.

Elizabeth, A., Applegate and Grivetti, L. 1997: Search for the competitive edge. A history of dietary fads and supplements. Symposium on nutrition and physical performance. A century of progress and tribute to the Modern Olympic Movement. *Journal of Nutrition* 127(55): 857S-886S.

Eleanor Noss Whitney Sharon Rady Rolfer, 7th Den, Understanding Nutrition 1993: West Publishing Company, St. Paul. pp. 510-535, 111-146, 153-193, 196-229, 344-387, 429-505.

Fujisawa Takuji, Kathleen Mulligan, Leslie Wada, Laurince Schumacher Jacques Riby and Norman Kretchmer 1993: The effect of exercise on fructose absorption. *American Journal of Clinical Nutrition* 58: 75-79.

Garrow, J. S. and James, W. P. T., 1993: *Human Nutrition and Dietetics 9th* Edn. Exercise Sport and Athletics. Longman Group U. K. Publisher Churchill Livingstone, pp. 409-441.

Gisolfi, C. V., Summers, R. W., Schedl, H. P., Bleiler, T. L., 1992: Intestinal water absorption from select carbohydrate solutions in humans, *Journal of Applied Physiology* 73 : 2142-2150.

Goodman, L. S. and Gilman , A., 1975: *The Pharmacological Basis of Therapeutics* 5th edn. N. Y. Macmillan Publishing Company, pp. 137-373.

Hanley, D. F., 1979: *Drug use and abuse*. In strauss R. H. ed. Sports Medicine and Physiology Philadelphia W.B., Saunders Company, 396-404.

Hargreaves, M., Costill, D. L., Fink, W. J., King D. S., 1987: Effect of pre-exercise carbohydrate feedings on endurance cycling performance, *Medical Science of Sports Exercise,* 19:33-36.

Hargreaves, M., *Carbohydrates and Exercise, in Foods, Nutrition and Sports Performance. An International Scientific Consus,* Eds C. Williams and J.T. Devlin, London: E & FN Spon, 1992, pp. 19-33.

Haymes, E. M., 1983: Protein, *Vitamins and Iron in: Williams* M.H. (ed), Ergogenic Aids in Sports. Champaign I. L: Human Kinetics Publishers Inc. 90-96.

Holloszy and Khort, 1996: Substrate metabolism during exercise. *Annual Reviews on Nutrition,* 121-137.

Howald and Segessers B., 1975: Ascorbic acid and athletic performance. Annals of the New York Academy of Sciences, 258:458-464.

Hortman, D. H., 1972: *Nutrition in Ergogenic Aids and Muscular Performance,* Academic Press, New York, pp. 343-365.

Hunt, J. N. and Spurrell, W. R., 1951: *The Pattern of Emptying of the Human Stomach.* Journal of Physiology, London, 113:157-168.

Jakovlev, N. N., 1975: *Vitamin Requirements in Athlete Nutrition Warsaw,* 22-24, October, 1975, Polish Sports Federation, p. 33.

James, F., Hickson, Ira Wolinsky James, M., Pivarnik Elizabeth A.,Newman B. S., Josehph, F., Itak and John, E., and Stockton, 1987: Nutrition Research, 7: 27-34.

Jensen, C. R. and Fisher, A. G., 1979: Scientific bases of athletic conditioning 2nd Philadelphia Lea and Febiger.

Jokl, E., 1968: *Notes on doping in Jokl* E and Jokl P(Ed.), Exercise and attitude Basal S. Karger.

Karen Eich Drummond, 2 ND den, Nutrition for the Food Service Professional 1994, Van Nostrand Reinhold—A division of International, Thomson Publishing Inc. New York.

Koivisto Veikko, Sirkka Lissa Karonen and Esko A., Nikkila, 1981: *Carbohydrate Ingestion before Exercise: Comparison of Glucose, Fructose and Sweet Placebo.* Journal of Applied Physiology,Respiratory Environmental Exercise Physiology, 51(4), 783-787.

Kovisto, V., Harkonen M., Groop P. H., 1985: Glycogen depletion during prolonged exercise:influence of glucose, fructose or placebo. Journal of Applied Physiology 58: 731-737.

Kreider, R. B., and Thompson, W. R., 1986: *Ketone Bodies and Ketosis in Exercise.* Ann Sports Med 2(4): 170.

Krogh and Lindhard, 1920: Relative value of fat and carbohydrate as source of muscular energy. *Biochemistry Journal,* 14: 290-363.

Lamb, D. R., Brodowicz, G. R., 1986: Optimal use of fluids of varying formulations to minimise exercise induced disturbances in homeostasis.

Levine, L., Evans, W., Cadarette B., Fisher E. and Bullen, B. A., 1983: Fructose and glucose ingestion and muscle glycogen use during submaximal exercise. Journal of Applied Physiology, *Respirotary Environmental Exercise Physiology,* 55(6):1767-1771.

Lindsay, M., Weight, Trimothy D., Nokes Dimitri Labadoris, John Graves, Peter Jacob and Peter Berman, 1988, Vitamin and Mineral status of trained Athletes including the effects of supplementation. *American Journal of Clinical Nutrition* 47:186-191.

Malhotra, M. S., Ramaswamy, S. S., Joseph, N. and Sen Gupta., J., 1972: Physiological assessment of Indian Athletes, Defence Institute of Physiology and Allied Sciences, Delhi Cannt, 103, Indian Journal of Physiological Pharmacology 16(1):55.

Maurice Jettle, Omer Pelletier Louise Parker and James, Thoden, 1978: The nutritional and metabolic effects of a carbohydrate-rich diet in a glycogen supercompensation training regimen. *American Journal of Clinical Nutrition* 31: 2140-48.

Mc Hugh, P. R. and Moron, T. H., 1979: Calories and gastric emptying a regulatory capacity with implications for feeding, *American Journal of Physiology* 236: R254-R260.

Mitchell, J. B., Costill D. L., Houmand, J.A., 1989: Gastric emptying influence of prolonged exercise and carbohydrate concentration. *Medical Science Sports Exercise*, 21:269-274.

Murray, R., Paul, G.L., Seifert, G. J., Eddy, D. E., Haleby, G. A., 1989: The effects of glucose, fructose and sucrose ingestion during exercise, *Medical Science Sports Exercise*, 21:275-82.

Narasinga Rao, B. S., 1996: Nutrient requirement of sports persons and athletes. *Proceedings of Nutrition Society of India* 43:79-103.

Nimmi Ittycheria John 2003——————————————————Food and Nutrition World——————————————————.

Okano, G., Takeda, H., Morita, Ikatoh, M., Muz Migake, S., 1988: Effect of pre-exercise fructose ingestion on endurance performance in fed man. Medicine and Science in Sports and Exercise 20:105-09.

Passmore, R., and Durnin, J.V.G.A., 1955: Physiol Rev. 35, 801.

Rasch, P. J. and Pierson, W. R., 1962: Effect of a protein dietary supplement on muscular strength and hypertrophy. *American Journal of Clinical Nutrition*, 11:530-32.

Sarah, H., Short and William, R. Short., 1983: Four year study of university athlete's dietary intake, *Journal of the American Dietetic Association* 82(6):632-45.

Satyanarayana, K., Rao, N. B. S., Rao, M. S. and Malhotra M.S., 1985: Recommended dietary intakes for Indian Sportsmen and Women. *National Institute of Nutrition*, Hyderabad.

Shapiro, H. and Stoner, E. K., 1968: Gastric temperature adaptation. *American Journal of Gastroenterology* 49: 391-404.

Shepherd, R., 1972 : Alive man, the physiology of physical activity. *Spring* Field, *Thomas.*

Shi X, Summers, R.W., Schedl, H.P., 1995: Effect of carbohydrate type and concentration and solution osmolality on water absorption, *Medical Science Sports Exercise in Press.*

Swaminathan, M., 1998: Nutrition of athletes. Essentials of Food and Nutrition, Vol. 1, Fundamental Aspects 2nd Edn. Bangalore Printing and Publishing Company ltd., Bangalore, p. 607.

Tremblay, A., Boilaro F., Berton, M. I., Bessette, H. and Roberge, A. G., 1984. The effect of riboflavin supplementation on the nutritional status and performance of elite swimmers, *Nutrition Research,* 4:201-08.

Ulmark, R., 1963: The dangers of doping, *Journal of Sports Medicine and Physical Fitness* 3:248.

Usha, Chandrashekar, Sakthivevel, A. and Sujatha, R., 1988: Nutritional Status of athletes and impact of dietary modification on their athletic performance. *The Indian Journal of Nutrition and Dietetics,* 25:176-181.

Usha, Chandrashekar and Shantipriya, S., 1989: Nutritional Profiles and Impact of dietary modification on the athletic performance. *The Indian Journal of Nutrition and Dietetics,* 26: 279-287.

Vaijayanthi, Kanabur and Kamini Devi (2005): Journal of Food Science and Technology 42(5):460-65.

Vukovich, M. D., Costill, D. L., Hickey, M. S., Trappe, S. W., Cole K. J., Fink, W. J., 1993: Effect of fat emulsion infusion and fat on muscle glycogen utilization during cycle exercise. *Journal of Applied Physiology,* 75:1513-1508.

Williams, M., 1974: Drugs and Athletic Performance Spring Field Thomas In: Asma Sultana 1993 Impact of dietary modification and nutrition education on athletic performance M Sc Thesis. Andhra Pradesh Agricultural University. Hyderabad, p. 116.

Williams, M. H., 1982: Vitamin, iron and calcium supplementation effect on human physical performance In: Haskell, W., Scala, J., Whitam, J., Nutrition and athletic performance Palo Alto, C. A. Bull Publishing Company, pp:106-153.

Wright, E. D., 1985: *Carbohydrate Nutrition and Exercise.* Clin. Nutr, 7(1),18.

Index